asthma-free
naturally

everything you need
to know to take control
of your asthma

asthma-free
naturally

Patrick McKeown

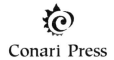

Conari Press

Published in 2008 by Conari Press,
an imprint of Red Wheel/Weiser, LLC
With offices at:
500 Third Street, Suite 230
San Francisco, CA 94107
www.redwheelweiser.com

10 9 8 7 6 5 4 3 2 1

First published by Asthma Care, Furbo, Co. Galway 2003
Published by HarperThorsons, an imprint of HarperCollinsPublishers,
in 2005

Illustrations by Manish Shah of www.globalsolutionsindia.com

Library of Congress Cataloging-in-Publication Data available upon
request

ISBN: 978-1-57324-372-8

Printed and bound in China

contents

'Without mastering breathing, nothing can be mastered.'

– P.D. Ouspensky

acknowledgements

Special thanks to editor Angela Doyle and Paper Tigers who wove together 60,000 words into perfect sequence according to a tight deadline.

I am extremely grateful to Liam and Anne Maher and family for their continued support and encouragement throughout every step of Asthma Care. Thanks also to Ronan Maher and Maurice Curtin who helped proofread and edit the first drafts of this book.

I am also deeply thankful to Bill Power for his early editing of the manuscript, his very helpful insights, his sense of humour and feedback.

Special thanks to Kevin Kelly, who provided me with an accurate expectation of the trials and tribulations of writing this book, from the first written word to final completion.

To those people who willingly gave up their time to be interviewed on RTE and TV3 and the Irish media, thank you so much for helping to create greater awareness of this therapy. A special thanks to Yvonne and Lorcan Cooke, Elizabeth Mullins, Shane Fitzgibbon, Sue Emerson, Liam Lawlor (not the politician), Maura Coyle, Aoife Quinn, Anne Wilson, Jean McConnell and Peter Moran.

I am deeply indebted to the Irish media for reporting on the merits of correct volume breathing for asthmatics and in particular to the work of Anthony Garvey and Kevin Murphy.

Many thanks to Carla Magliocco for managing operations on a day-to-day basis and for directing the future path of Asthma Care.

Other people who have helped me indirectly throughout the years and who deserve special recognition are Adrian Sisk, Alan Loughrey and Terry Clune.

Special thanks to Dr Andrey Novozhilov and Luidmilla Buteyko, my teachers, and to the greatest scientist of all time, the late Professor Konstantin Buteyko. Thank you for your undivided attention and for providing humanity with its greatest discovery to date.

To Sinead, the balance in my life, my partner and soul mate, thank you.

Finally, I would like to express my love and gratitude to my mother, father and brothers, without whom this book would not exist.

introduction

This book teaches you how to take control of your asthma safely and effectively without any side effects. The approach encompasses the Buteyko Clinic Method and instruction on diet, sleeping, physical activity and other lifestyle factors. I had chronic asthma for twenty years but since making these changes to my lifestyle, I have been completely asthma free.

The Buteyko (Bhew-tae-ko) Clinic Method is recognised by the Russian medical authorities. Not alone that, but it has been backed up by two independent scientific trials held in the Western world. The method has received widespread attention including a detailed debate in the UK House of Commons in July 2001. Evidence from thousands of people worldwide – who improved their lives forever by applying Buteyko breathing exercises – is also available.

This non-medical treatment is based on the life's work of Russian respiratory physiologist, Professor Konstantin Buteyko, who developed a programme of exercises to foster correct breathing. The Buteyko Clinic Method is based on bodily processes and not on a placebo effect.

There are three ways of controlling asthma. The first and most important is learning to breathe through the lungs' natural defence – the nose – combined with correct breathing. The second is living a life balanced by proper nutrition, regular exercise and relaxation. The third avenue is using preventative and relieving asthma medication.

Think of it as a three-way junction where you, the person with asthma, can choose the direction. The first two avenues are like the scenic routes: they're entirely natural, proven and improve overall health, but require personal commitment and an investment of time and energy. The third avenue is the one most often travelled by people like you but it never addresses the root cause of your breathing problem. The third avenue also involves taking chemicals which are alien to your body. Sooner or later, your body fights back or submits to the continuous use of powerful drugs.

I'm often told that people with asthma are fortunate to have such a wide range of medication available to them now, and I agree. We are fortunate. However, as a person with asthma myself, I feel that being dependent on medication for survival generates feelings of weakness and vulnerability. That being said, I always stress to my patients that medication, especially preventer medication, is very important, but that they should take enough to maintain control – no more and no less. Likewise, I advise patients to try to avoid situations that are likely to trigger an attack.

I was diagnosed with asthma as a child, a condition that worsened as I grew older until I discovered Buteyko Breathing through a newspaper article. I learned as much as I could, self-taught the techniques, and found myself gradually reducing the amount of medication I had to take to control my asthma.

When I experienced the impressive benefits of the Buteyko Method, I wondered why more people didn't know about it or how to apply it to their own lives. I decided to explore the possibility of training so that I could teach this beautiful and simple method to asthma sufferers like myself. I found out that I could enrol at the Buteyko Clinic of Moscow and, after many trials and tribulations, I started my training under Dr Andrey Novozhilov and Dr Luidmilla Buteyko. The Buteyko Clinic of Moscow was founded by Professor Konstantin Buteyko as a centre for the treatment and prevention of health problems. The Buteyko Clinic Method is used to describe the programme of breathing exercises as taught by the Buteyko Clinic of Moscow.

I was accredited by Professor Buteyko in March of 2002, and since this time, the knowledge I gained in Moscow has been complemented by my own research, by consulting with asthma specialists from different parts of the world, and by ongoing client contact throughout Ireland.

The simple question is: does it work? In a word: yes. Some patients achieve excellent results effortlessly, but with others it takes a little more time and determination. The success of this therapy for every patient depends on the patient's ability to put the theory into practice. There is no big mystery – this therapy is based on normal body processes. Scientific trials have shown clearly that the Buteyko Method can be one hundred per cent effective in the treatment of asthma.

The only real key to the effectiveness of the therapy is that individuals are prepared to set aside the necessary time to learn and practice the exercises.

I commend those of you who, on reading this book, will decide to make that effort. I can honestly say that your investment of time and energy will be gratifying, and that it will transform your life ... for the rest of your life.

I can hear you thinking that there's no such thing as a free lunch, and that there's always a catch. There is no catch this time. Once you learn how to control your own asthma, you are in charge of your own life and treatment. This therapy is about teaching you the skills to deal with your own asthma problem; my job is essentially to make myself redundant.

This book, written by a person with asthma for people with asthma, contains essential information to help you deal with your condition. Each exercise is a simplified version to make the contents as user-friendly as possible in the hope that you will be able to understand and appreciate this approach, and that you will be able to apply it practically to your own asthma problem.

Included is a special section for children who naturally will have difficulty understanding breathing patterns. Every child who comes to me is told how lucky he or she is to be learning a therapy as effective as this, a therapy that deals with what otherwise would be a life-long illness ... without medicine, tablets, hospital visits or injections.

At our clinics throughout the Republic of Ireland and Northern Ireland, patients receive practical help and advice and our training exercises are designed to suit the individual needs of each person. My clinics also address lifestyle factors such as correct breathing during physical activity, diet, sleeping, stress and much more. Clinics are a very useful way of exchanging information and answering any questions participants may have.

Feedback from those who attend our clinics has been extremely helpful in furthering my own knowledge of asthma, in developing the content of future clinics, and also in the writing of this book.

There's another simple question you may have at this point: why is the Buteyko method not better known? That's a good question, and one to which I don't have a clear answer. Looking at the current situation openly, however, one of the most striking features is that medical research is mainly funded by pharmaceutical companies, in one form or another. Asking the pharmaceutical industry to fund research into a method such as Buteyko – with its non-medication approach – is perhaps like asking turkeys to vote in favour of Christmas. The usual answer is that there has been insufficient research for authoritative judgements to be made.

If a non-medication approach to asthma such as the Buteyko Method achieved widespread acceptance in Ireland, there would be massive savings in the national health budget. Given the potential for savings, the Department of Health should be interested in commissioning or supporting research into the method. To date, there has been no indication of any awareness of this potential by the Department.

My main aim is to help people overcome their asthma-related problems by using the Buteyko Clinic Method and lifestyle changes. When enough people have experienced the benefits, I hope that public opinion might have enough leverage on medical authorities to encourage them to assess Professor Buteyko's method with an open mind. If that happens, then at least there will be a long-delayed debate on the subject.

I am open to any comments, suggestions or criticism which you may have regarding this book. Constant feedback from my patients has already improved my understanding of asthma and my ability to help people.

All this therapy involves is a commitment to observation of breathing and practice of simple breathing exercises, plus a reasonably well-balanced lifestyle. The reward is freedom. The prize is freedom from asthma.

I wish you every success in applying this tried and tested method developed by an extraordinary Russian doctor.

Patrick McKeown BA MA (TCD) Dip. Buteyko (Moscow)

asthma for beginners

'No matter what treatment you avail of and no matter what medications you take for your asthma, as long as you continue to overbreathe, you will continue to have asthma.'

This book is about taking control of your asthma safely and without the need for medication. You will read about how I transformed myself from an acute asthmatic with a permanent illness requiring daily drug intake – and hospitalisation from time to time – to a virtual non-asthmatic who is totally free from asthma symptoms, attacks ... and medication.

You may not believe that this scenario is real. It is. I achieved it and any asthmatic can achieve it too. This non-medical treatment is based on the life's work of Russian respiratory physiologist, Professor Konstantin Buteyko, who developed a programme of exercises to foster correct breathing. The Buteyko Method is based on bodily processes, not on a placebo or any other effect. All persons with asthma can learn it and use it; the method is very simple, will entail minimum disruption to your life, and you will notice an improvement in as little as seven days. Like I said, you still may not believe this scenario is real. Believe it now.

Asthma was diagnosed when I was very young. Initially my condition was mild and consisted of just occasional wheezing and breathlessness. The treatment consisted of using an Intal inhaler. I only had an attack occasionally, so my asthma didn't really disrupt my life.

When I reached the age of ten, my asthma deteriorated a little so I was prescribed a Ventolin inhaler which guaranteed me immediate relief from the symptoms. I had to take a Uniphyiulum tablet each night as well. At the time, just one puff of Ventolin dealt with any breathing difficulty I experienced. My asthma was under control.

With the best of intentions, our doctor told my mother that children with asthma very often 'grow out of it' during their teenage years. Time and time again, I was assured that this should happen, and it offered a ray of hope for me, but this hope was never realised. As I grew into adulthood, the dose needed to maintain control of my asthma increased. One puff of Ventolin per day was no longer enough. Soon I was taking two, five, eight and even ten puffs a day. My lifestyle during my school and college years didn't help, but I had my Ventolin inhaler to help me overcome any problems so I wasn't too concerned about it.

One weekend, when I was in my early twenties, I was brought to James Connolly Memorial Hospital with an asthma attack, and I was told that I was being treated for acute asthma. Two weeks of large doses of oral steroids later, I returned home.

As the years passed, the amount of medication I needed continued to increase. There was no great discussion about this with my doctor, nor any indication that the amount of drugs I needed would ever decline. It seemed to me that I was going steadily downhill, and I became gradually more concerned about the effect that the increasing levels of medication might be having on my general health and well-being.

Many people with asthma can relate to this summary of the steady progression of the condition. What starts off as an occasional wheeze soon develops into continuous symptoms; while one puff of medication deals with symptoms in the early stages, dependency on medication increases remorselessly.

Over time, my asthma developed into a seriously debilitating condition that prevented me from taking part in sport and outdoor activities. I always avoided opportunities to play a match or work out in the gym. The physical limitations were one thing, but the stigma attached to me because of my asthma was another. I had 'weak lungs', and I was not as physically strong as lads of my age. Initially, when I was very young, I thought it was cool to carry an inhaler – it was a neat gadget that made me different – but as I got older it labelled me in a way I didn't like. When I realised this, in the succeeding years I always tried to take my inhaler when there was no-one else around, for all the world like a secret drinker.

While I grappled with the daily realities of having asthma, there were two unanswered questions at the back of my mind. When is this ever going to stop? Why am I so inadequate that I have to take daily doses of drugs merely to function normally? I was turning myself into a victim, but these are common questions that will be familiar to many asthma sufferers. The questions may not be voiced openly because complaining will do little to change what may seem like an unalterable reality, but they are still very real concerns.

The first indication I had that there was a viable alternative to taking a Ventolin inhaler in secret arrived in my early twenties, when I happened upon an article in the *Irish Independent* newspaper about a breathing therapy developed by a Russian professor which seemed to be effective in helping people with asthma. Over the years, I had already tried acupuncture, Chinese herbs, deep-breathing exercises and indeed any other therapy that I felt might help. When Buteyko Breathing was featured in a magazine article shortly afterwards, I decided to find out more.

I started my search for knowledge by contacting Buteyko practitioners from around the world via the Internet. I learned as much as possible about the application of the therapy and I purchased the limited publications and videos available at the time. I taught myself the technique, used it intensively, and I was pleasantly surprised at the rapid effect it had on my asthma. Intuitively, I felt that I understood the significance of Professor Buteyko's work ... even before I began applying it.

In a matter of months, my asthma improved so dramatically that I could reduce my medication intake significantly. As my condition continued to improve and my medication intake continued to decrease, I felt that for the first time in my life my asthma was under control. The bonus for me was that I had achieved this myself. My days of secretly puffing Ventolin were behind me.

Elixir of life

Take a breath now, and think about it carefully. Breathing is the elixir of life. More than that, breathing is life. We humans can live without water for days and without food for weeks, but we cannot live without air for more than a few minutes. Think about how we Westerners view food and water: we know that the quantity and quality of food and water we consume determines our state of health. We know that having too little means starvation or dehydration, and that too much leads to obesity and other health problems.

Why then does the quantity and quality of our breathing receive so little attention? Surely breathing, which is so immediately essential to life, must meet certain conditions? Why have other cultures, particularly in the Eastern world, recognised the importance of correct breathing to health for thousands of years, when we clearly don't?

What is asthma?

There is no universally accepted definition of asthma. The *Concise Oxford Dictionary* describes it as 'a disease of respiration characterised by difficult breathing, cough etc.'. Any good medical book will describe it in more technical terms but 'difficult breathing' is the part with which any asthma sufferer is familiar, even if it varies from mildly uncomfortable to life-threatening. Asthma is news now. There was a dramatic increase in the condition in the late twentieth century to the extent that an estimated 100 to 150 million people in the world are now affected by it, but it is not a recent phenomenon.[1]

The term 'asthma' is a Greek translation of gasping or panting, and the problem was treated as far back as 2000 BC by Chinese doctors with the herb Ma Huang. The first known recording of the symptoms was about 3,500 years ago in an ancient Egyptian manuscript called *Ebers Papyrus*. Throughout the ages, asthma has received varying degrees of attention; the symptoms and their accompanying anxiety have been described by many prominent historical figures, including the famous Greek physician, Hippocrates.

Over the centuries, there has been an assortment of different theories about the causes of asthma, and so an eclectic range of remedies has been advised, including horse riding, strong coffee, tobacco, faith healing, chloroform and even drinking the blood of owls in wine, as practised by the ancient Romans. Van Helmont who lived in the early part of the seventeenth century claimed that asthma was epilepsy of the lungs due to the sudden and unpredictable nature of an attack. Based on his own experience of asthma, English physician Thomas Willis said that 'the blood boils', and that 'there is scarce anything more sharp or terrible than the fits thereof'.

It was not until the eighteenth century that Lavoisier provided the first real account of the functioning of the lungs, thereby providing the basis of modern-day understanding of the respiratory system. Prior to this, it was commonly believed that air was drawn into the lungs to cool the body. Lavoisier's contribution was that air is drawn in to be converted to energy by the metabolism, and that carbon dioxide and heat are produced as end products of the process. Lavoisier's work recognised that oxygen is essential to sustaining life.

Asthma now affects more people throughout the world, particularly in more developed countries, than at any other time in evolution. It inflicts greater economic and social damage in Western Europe than either TB or HIV, according to the World Health Organisation's (WHO) April 2002 report on the links between ill health in children and the deteriorating environment.

The position in selected developed countries may be summed up as follows (all figures are approximate):

	Asthma Diagnosed (millions)	Population (millions)	%
USA[2]	20	285	7.0
UK[3]	5.1	60	8.5
Australia[4]	2	19	10.5
Ireland[5]	0.3	3.9	7.7

According to the 1998 International Study of Asthma and Allergies in Childhood (ISAAC), the countries with the highest twelve-month incidence of asthma were the UK, Australia, New Zealand and the Republic of Ireland followed by North, Central and South America. The same report found that the lowest rates were in centres in several Eastern European countries, followed by Indonesia, Greece, China, Taiwan, Uzbekistan, India and Ethiopia. Other studies show that the rate of asthma among rural Africans who migrate to cities and adopt a more 'western' urbanised lifestyle increases dramatically. According to the UCB Institute of Allergy in Belgium, the incidence of asthma in Western Europe has doubled in the last ten years.[1]

In the Western world, asthma crosses all class, race, geography and gender boundaries. Although it causes persistent symptoms among seventy per cent of all people diagnosed with it, asthma causes only minor discomfort to the majority. In fact, some of the most influential people of our time in all walks of life were asthmatic, including Russian Tzar Peter the Great, actors Liza Minnelli, Jason Alexander and Elizabeth Taylor, revolutionary Che Guevara, and former US presidents John F Kennedy, Calvin Coolidge and Theodore Roosevelt. All these have lived life to the full or are still living it.

What are the symptoms?

So what is asthma and what are the symptoms? The condition consists of inflammation, tightening and swelling of the airways in the respiratory system, resulting in obstruction of the flow of air to and from the lungs. The symptoms of asthma include breathlessness, wheezing, coughing and chest tightness. Sufferers may also have a blocked nose, frequent colds and hay fever, or rhinitis. The symptoms and their severity are peculiar to the individual, and they vary from season to season and according to the individual's susceptibility to a wide range of triggers.

An 'asthma attack' is the term used to describe an episode of breathing difficulty. In some cases, this may follow exposure to a specific trigger, such as dust, pollen, or certain

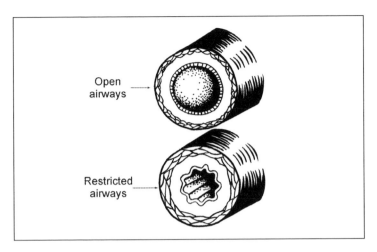

Open airways

Restricted airways

Airways narrowing

foods. In other cases there appears to be no particular trigger. Some people have a cough and no wheeze, while others may have a wheeze and very little coughing, but each case is accompanied by some level of breathing difficulty. Symptoms may occur periodically, on a day-to-day or season-to-season basis, or they may be more or less continuous.

A 'trigger' is something that makes asthma worse. The most common triggers include (in alphabetical order): allergies; cigarette smoking (and cigarette smoke for non-smokers); colds and flu; cold air; dust mites; exercise under certain circumstances; moulds; noxious fumes; pollens; stress, and weather types such as fog and damp. In some instances an asthma attack may be triggered by a combination of catalysts. Anxiety can be caused by the variations on the asthma theme, particularly where a child is involved. Sometimes, there may be confusion between doctor and patient when a diagnosis is being made.

There is also a wide variety in the symptoms of asthma. The following is a list of those most commonly experienced by sufferers.

✦ **Wheeze**
This is a high pitched whistling sound produced when air is forced through narrowed airways. If you blow through a Biro pen when the ink refill is removed, the sound is similar.

✦ **Breathlessness**
This is the feeling of not being able to take in enough air. There is a need to breathe out while, at the same time, a compulsion to breathe in. If this symptom develops to an extreme level it can be frightening for the sufferer and very distressing for those close to him or her.

✦ **Coughing**
This may be either a repetitive dry cough or a cough with phlegm, often occurring during the night or early morning. Repetitive coughing can put a strain on the heart and drives sputum deeper into the lungs. Patients with this symptom may feel like they are on a conveyor belt: the more they cough, the more they feel the need to cough again.

✦ **Chest tightness**
Trapped air in the lungs generates a feeling that the chest is over inflated. This is often described as someone squeezing or sitting on one's chest.

✦ Frequent yawning

When asthma symptoms are at their worst, sleep is interrupted by difficult periods of breathing which contributes to tiredness.

Non-asthmatics can, of course, observe these symptoms, but they will not appreciate the feelings of tension, panic, uncertainty and helplessness which accompany them, particularly when the asthmatic struggles to breathe. If you are not an asthmatic, imagine trying to breathe while a pillow is being pressed firmly over your face. That feeling you imagine is the feeling someone with asthma has during an attack. In your case, the imaginary pillow can be easily removed to allow you to breathe effortlessly; for an asthmatic, the remedy is not so simple.

Given the variety of symptoms and their severity, diagnosing a condition that has no commonly accepted definition is not an exact science. Many asthma symptoms are also the symptoms of other conditions, such as chronic bronchitis or bronchiectasis, for example. Diagnosis has to take into account the chronic nature of asthma and the constriction of the airways due to inflammation by various cells and chemicals. Generally, diagnosis of asthma is based on the following factors.

✦ History of the patient

This includes establishing if the patient has experienced asthma symptoms while at rest, during exercise or after exposure to a known trigger.

✦ **Lung function tests**

The peak flow meter measures the maximum speed at which the patient can exhale air in one second. A person with asthma usually produces a lower reading, and, generally speaking, a more inconsistent range of results than a person who doesn't suffer from the condition. Spirometry measures both the speed and volume of air which is exhaled with each breath, thereby providing additional airway obstruction information.

✦ **Effect of reliever or steroidal medication**

In part, diagnosis of asthma is based on the effects of medication, and whether or not it leads to a temporary reversal of symptoms. Other conditions which demonstrate common asthma-type symptoms, such as emphysema, include irreversible airway obstruction.

✦ **Provocation test**

The patient inhales a broncho-constricting agent, such as histamine or methacholine. The airways of people with asthma are far more responsive to inhalation of these substances; agents like these will provoke more extensive narrowing of air passages in people with asthma.

✦ **Skin tests to determine allergies**

A number of common allergens are selected, such as dust mites, pollen or animal dander. One at a time, the allergens are placed on the forearm, and the skin is then gently pierced to allow the substances to penetrate. After fifteen minutes, the skin surrounding this spot may

develop a small rash. While this test is not always conclusive, the presence of a rash and the size of the weal indicate an allergy to a specific substance.

+ **Chest x-ray**

X-ray is used to rule out other respiratory diseases in a
person who has the symptoms of severe chronic asthma.
X-ray charts show irreversible damage to the airways, and
this aids the diagnoses of other respiratory disorders.

Your respiratory system

Before you commence breathing retraining, it is important
for you to have a basic understanding of the roles played by
the respiratory system and carbon dioxide in your body. Your
respiratory system consists of the parts of your body used for
the delivery of oxygen from the atmosphere to your cells and
tissues, and for transporting the carbon dioxide produced in
your tissues back into the atmosphere. If cells and tissues are
to function properly – if you are to live – your body needs the
atmosphere's oxygen. Your nose, mouth, pharynx, larynx,
trachea, bronchi and lungs are all part of your respiratory
system.

Part of your airways is your nose and mouth. Through
them, air enters your body and flows down a flexible tube
called the trachea. This tube eventually divides into two
branches called bronchi: one branch enters the left lung and
the other branch enters the right. Within your lungs, the
bronchi further subdivide into an estimated twenty-five

smaller branches called bronchioles. The bronchioles run
into alveolar ducts and at the end are small air sacs called
alveoli.

Look at it another way. Imagine an upside-down tree.
The trachea is the trunk; at the top of the trunk are the two
large branches of the bronchi. From each of these large
branches grow the smaller branches of the bronchioles. At
the end of each smaller branch are the 'leaves', the round
balloon-shaped sacs called alveoli.

When you breathe in, air enters through your nose or
mouth and flows into the trachea, the bronchi, bronchioles
and eventually alveoli. The grape-like alveoli – after which
they are named – are surrounded by tiny blood channels
called capillaries. Oxygen enters the blood by passing
through a very thin barrier between the capillaries and air
sacs. It is then carried by what is called haemoglobin within

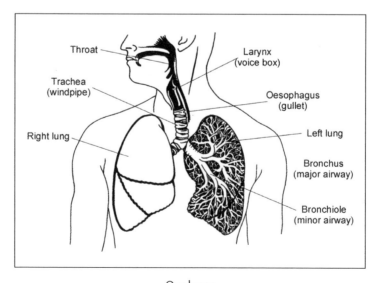

Our lungs

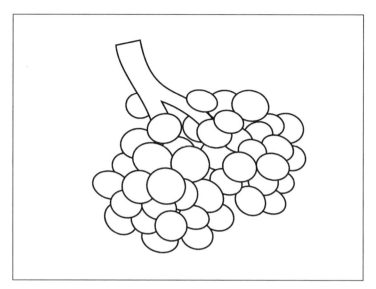

A close-up of Alveoli (air sacs)

the blood to tissues and cells. There are approximately three hundred million alveoli in the lungs, each of which is surrounded by tiny blood vessels.

To put this huge number in context, think of Wimbledon and imagine a tennis court. The area of contact between your alveoli and blood capillaries is equivalent to the size of a tennis court; as you can imagine, this massive area provides scope for an efficient transfer of oxygen from the air to your blood. Carbon dioxide is produced as an end product of the process of breaking down the fats and carbohydrates that you eat, and this gas is brought by your venous blood vessels to your lungs where the excess is exhaled. Crucially, part of your body's quotient of carbon dioxide is retained when you exhale, and correct breathing results in the required amount of carbon dioxide being retained in your lungs.

There are two main aspects to the way you breathe. Your *rate* is the number of breaths you take in one minute and your *volume* is the amount of air drawn into your lungs. Although the two are separate, one generally influences the other. The volume of air we inhale and exhale is measured in litres, and measurements are usually taken over one minute. In conventional medicine, the accepted number of breaths a healthy person takes in one minute is ten to twelve, with each breath drawing in a volume of 500 millilitres. In a full minute, this provides the body with a total volume of five to six litres. If a person is breathing at a higher rate of twenty breaths, for example, then the volume will also be higher, and vice-versa. To visualise this amount of air, imagine how much air would be contained in a two-litre soft drink bottle.

Where to now?

So, now you know how the respiratory system works, and you or someone close to you has been diagnosed with asthma. Where to now? A lifetime of drug therapy? Or a proven, natural, physiology-based way of reversing what can be a debilitating condition?

A new beginning is emerging in the treatment of asthma, aimed at getting to the root cause of the problem. By addressing the cause rather than the symptoms that are the effect, sufferers finally have the ability to be able to take control of their own condition, naturally and permanently. This new beginning is based on the life's work of Russian scientist, Professor Konstantin Buteyko. Before we can begin to look at how you can change your own life, we must take a brief look at his.

Over four decades, Professor Buteyko completed pioneering work on illnesses which develop as a result of breathing a volume of air greater than the body requires. His work provided mankind with probably the greatest discovery to date in the field of medicine.

As a medical student, Konstantin observed hundreds of sick patients, and realised that their breathing was closely related to the extent of their illness. The greater the volume of air which a patient inhaled, the greater their sickness, he discovered. This relationship was so precise that he was able to predict accurately the exact time when ill patients would pass away.

Through his research, he devised a breathing programme for his patients based on reducing the amount of air that passed through their lungs. When each patient applied reduced breathing, all their bodily functions including pulse, volume of breathing per minute and blood pressure were monitored. The resulting data enabled him to refine and improve his method. Buteyko's theory is based on the life force of any organism: breathing.

Like many other revolutionary findings, it can often take many years before a discovery is acknowledged and incorporated into everyday practice. Take Professor Lister, for example. He discovered that many illnesses such as sepsis could be passed by the contaminated hands of a doctor to a patient. Lister tested his hypothesis by disinfecting his hands before each operation and this resulted in a decrease in the death rate of his patients. It took many years for this discovery to be accepted by the medical community; it was only really accepted when patients' relatives started demanding that doctors disinfect their hands before operating.

Although research conducted in Russia in 1962 proved unequivocally the soundness of Buteyko's method, it was not until 1983 that the Committee on Inventions and Discoveries formally acknowledged his work. This recognition was backdated to January 29th, 1962. That backdating alone begs the question: if Konstantin Buteyko's discovery had been acknowledged earlier, how many more ill people would have been helped?

The first trials held in the Western world were at the Mater Hospital in Brisbane in 1995. After three months, the Buteyko group had seventy per cent less symptoms, ninety per cent less need for reliever medication and forty-nine per cent less need for steroids. Furthermore, those who corrected their breathing the most reduced their symptoms and need for medication the most. An article published in *Australian Doctor* on April 7th, 1995 was headed '*Doctors gasp at Buteyko success*'.

A second trial was conducted at Gisborne Hospital, New Zealand in 2003 and published in the New Zealand Medical Journal. After six months, the Buteyko group showed an 85 per cent reduced need for reliever medication and 50 per cent reduced need for inhaled steroid.

In the forty-odd years since Buteyko's discovery, it has improved the health and saved the lives of many thousands of people. Now that his enlightening revelation is becoming better known in the Western world, it will improve the health and save the lives of many more. You could be one of them.

how is your breathing?

'Habit is either the best of servants or the worst of masters.'

– Nathaniel Emmons

For the vast majority of people, breathing is an everyday fact of life which occurs on a subconscious level. It is something that is all too often taken for granted – until there's a problem. Yet breathing is the most important physiological function you can exercise control over and this is something that can easily be achieved through increased attention, observation and will-power. With practice both the rate and volume of breathing can be changed for the better and the only prerequisite is to be aware of the existing breathing pattern.

Claude Lum, a noted physician at Papworth University hospital, Cambridge, described hyperventilation, or over-breathing, as a bad habit that has the effect of lowering carbon dioxide levels. It is only necessary to look at examples such as smoking to realise that bad habits are easy to acquire – and not quite so easy to lose. Changing a habit of a lifetime can initially cause disruption to a daily routine and focus attention on the change that is to be made.

While in extreme cases the fight to combat a bad habit can consume every waking minute, acquiring a good habit can inspire a new wave of self-confidence. Once the new habit has been acquired, even one that requires enormous self-discipline and a large helping of patience, it quickly becomes very easy to live with and can help boost self-esteem and self-belief. The investment of time, effort and concentration in the short term will ensure a reward of positive long-term results.

Making the change to a reduced volume of breathing should be treated as simply acquiring a good habit – one that will reap untold health benefits. Ultimately the benefits can include the complete recovery of an individual with asthma.

Many of Professor Buteyko's patients who were taught the Buteyko Method remained completely free from symptoms of asthma thirty years later. It was as a result of pressure placed on the Soviet authorities by those who recovered that independent trials into Professor Buteyko's method were conducted. The results of the trials brought about the full recognition and acceptance of the Buteyko system in the Soviet Union.

What is overbreathing?

First, let's take a quick look at what overbreathing is, and why we do it in the first place. Clinically, overbreathing is known as hyperventilation; put simply, it means breathing more air than the body needs. The standard volume of normal breathing for a healthy adult is three to six litres of air per minute.

Scientific research conducted by Professor Buteyko over three decades, along with scientific trials at the Mater Hospital in Brisbane in 1995 demonstrated that people with asthma breathe a volume of ten to twenty litres per minute between attacks, and over twenty litres during an attack.

Overbreathing causes a loss of carbon dioxide from the lungs. This is not a problem if it occurs only for a short time, because breathing will reduce afterwards to restore the carbon dioxide levels. However, breathing more air than we need over a period of time – and time can mean hours, weeks, months or even years – will result in the day-to-day levels of carbon dioxide remaining low constantly. Our respiratory centre becomes accustomed to or fixed at these lower levels of carbon dioxide and determine them to be 'correct'. Our respiratory centre will therefore instruct us to overbreathe to maintain these low levels of carbon dioxide even though the rest of our bodily organs and tissues are suffering.

Carbon dioxide is very important for normal bodily functioning (for a more detailed explanation, see Appendix 1), it is logical to assume that the body must have some way to prevent losing it. Narrowing of the airways is caused by inflammation, by constriction of smooth muscle and by increased mucus secretion, and is a natural defence mechanism to help maintain the carbon dioxide level. In a person with asthma, this defence mechanism activates when the carbon dioxide level declines too much. Overbreathing also causes cooling and drying of the airways, two effects that have been recognised to play a role in producing asthma symptoms (for a more detailed explanation, see Appendix 2).

People with asthma are better off than anyone else who overbreathes because they are equipped with an instant defence mechanism to prevent the loss of carbon dioxide. People who do not have this defence mechanism suffer from many of the diseases of civilisation for which there is no cure. It is worth noting that before 1900, people who had asthma often lived longer than the rest of the population and that death from asthma was unknown. *'Having asthma generally meant having a long life free from many diseases, but nobody could explain why asthma prevented other diseases or why asthmatics lived longer than other people,'* Professor Buteyko noted. At the end of 19th century, Professor of Medicine at Oxford University Sir William Osler, wrote in his *Principles and Practice of Medicine* textbook: *'We have no knowledge of the morbid anatomy of true asthma. Death during the attack is unknown.'*

Overbreathing resulting from modern living is the cause of breathing-related diseases. Hyperventilation is not just a result of asthma, hyperventilation is the main contributor of asthma.

Professor Buteyko believes that genetic predisposition determines which illnesses people develop from overbreathing. As a result, each person who hyperventilates or overbreathes is affected individually, based on hereditary factors.

Symptoms of hyperventilation

Some of the symptoms of hyperventilation affect:

+ **The respiratory system** in the form of wheezing, breathlessness, coughing, chest tightness, frequent yawning, snoring and sleep apnoea.
+ **The nervous system** in the form of a light-headed feeling, poor concentration, numbness, sweating, dizziness, vertigo, tingling of hands and feet, faintness, trembling and headache.
+ **The heart**, typically a racing heartbeat, pain in the chest region, and a skipping or irregular heartbeat.
+ **The mind**, including some degrees of anxiety, tension, depression, apprehension and stress.
+ **Other general symptoms** include mouth dryness, fatigue, bad dreams, nightmares, dry itchy skin, sweaty palms, increased urination such as bed wetting or regular visits to the bathroom during the night, diarrhoea, constipation, general weakness and chronic exhaustion.

Why do we overbreathe?

Earlier on, I explained that when we overbreathe permanently, the respiratory centre in the brain is trained to accept a lower level of carbon dioxide. There are many reasons why we overbreathe, although not all of them may apply to everyone. These factors are more prevalent in countries experiencing increasing modernisation and affluence, and that prevalence helps explain why there are such high incidences of asthma and other diseases of civilisation in the same countries.

Briefly, these factors include: incorrect eating habits; the belief that it is good to take 'big breaths'; stress; more home heating; wearing too much clothing; lack of physical exercise, and pollution. Each of these are explored in more detail in Appendix 1.

Benefits of reduced breathing

Reduced breathing due to what is called the Bohr effect leads to better oxygenation of all of the body's cells and tissues which in turn enables all the organs to function more efficiently. Almost everyone who has attended Asthma Care clinics in Ireland has reported not just a significant improvement in their asthma, but also an improvement in their general health and well-being.

In addition, they reported increased energy levels; less dependence on stimulants such as caffeine; increased calmness; reduced anxiety and normalisation of weight – all within a relatively short period of time. Chronic complaints such as headaches, constipation and spasmodic conditions – caused by incorrect breathing and dietary factors or as result of side effects from asthma related medication – were also gradually eliminated.

Breaking the overbreathing habit

As babies we instinctively know how to breathe using the diaphragm, with the tummy moving up and down with each breath. For the most part, the breathing volume matches the exact needs of the metabolism; this is how the human body was intended to function and results in good health.

Parents strive to protect their children, yet by becoming over-protective they often contribute to problems for their offspring later in life. Parents habitually tend to over-dress young children and live in rooms that are too warm or too stuffy, while the children can also be exposed to an unsuitable diet which includes too much sugar and too many sweets, chocolates and fizzy drinks to which they soon become accustomed. It is then a simple progression along a slippery slope to a diet high in junk food, artificial additives and sweeteners, sometimes before a child even starts school.

Children are often advised by many sources to 'take a deep breath'. However, in this situation the word 'deep' is used in the wrong context and a deep breath in this case is actually a 'big' breath – filling the lungs but not using the diaphragm. So what are the necessary steps to break this habit?

✦ Step One
Acknowledge the bad habit – in this case overbreathing – and the reason why it is a bad habit. It is at this stage that the correct method of breathing is learned as well as the various ways of redressing the incorrect approach to breathing.

✦ Step Two

Often it is not until the breathing pattern has been corrected that it comes to light that it was incorrect in the first place. Therefore the solution lies in detecting the problem before it has even occurred. This pattern of detection and correction, caused by slipping back into bad habits, may continue for some time. Eventually, perhaps after much trial and error, becoming aware of the breathing pattern at an earlier stage can prevent overbreathing.

Psychologists claim that, with the correct attention and discipline, a bad habit can be broken and a new and better habit instilled in just 21 days. However, when it comes to learning a new way of breathing a little more time is required as the body becomes accustomed to a fundamental change in something as basic and essential as breathing. In reality, the time it takes is insignificant when compared with the benefits accruing from correct breathing.

✦ Step Three

With both time and effort good breathing should become routine, after all practice makes perfect. Eventually the good habit becomes like second nature and requires no conscious effort. Sticking to the better breathing routine will then require only intermittent attention to confirm the breathing is correct. The effort and discipline committed to learning this method of breathing will now pay off; this is a time to feel good.

Basic breath retraining

There are three basic steps towards breath retraining.

✦ Step One

Become very aware of your breathing. Feel, watch and listen to your breathing as much as you can during the day, paying particular attention to what causes you to take big breaths.

Ask yourself some questions. Is your breathing a still, silent activity or does it involve large inhalations and body movements? Are you going about your daily activities with your mouth open? Do you take a big breath as you stand up from your chair or before talking? Do you heave big sighs, yawn or sniff regularly? Do you wake in the night or early morning with a dry mouth? Is your nose blocked when you wake or do you wake feeling that you have not had a good night's sleep?

Only when you have become aware of your bad breathing can you take steps to correct it. During our clinics, we outline people's breathing traits. More often than not they are totally unaware of these and while some people find them alarming, more often most find them quite amusing.

Awareness of our own incorrect breathing can also be increased by observing other people who are perhaps breathing with their mouths open, panting when shopping, or at bus stops; it is also possible to notice a person's breathing characteristics over the telephone. Even though all of these people may seem to enjoy good health, many of those who have bad breathing actions may already have or are likely to develop health problems in the future.

✦ Step Two

Learn to breathe through your nose. Breathing through your nose at all times is the correct and only way to breathe.

The immortal message that 'the pint of plain is your only man' was brought to us by Flann O'Brien. However for those with asthma, nasal breathing is your only man, accompanied by the correct volume of breathing that will be discussed later on.

Some people seem to spend most of their lives with a blocked nose and many have tried, without success, every nasal spray and therapy on the market. In this book those very people will be taught an effective exercise for unblocking the nose in a matter of minutes. This will be the first step on the road to permanent and comfortable nasal breathing.

✦ Step Three

It has already been explained how the respiratory centre can accept a low level of carbon dioxide as the norm, despite the stress it may place on various organs. All the breathing exercises featured in this book involve breathing less air than the body has become accustomed to. Over time this helps reset the respiratory system to accept the higher levels of carbon dioxide that it really should have. Remember, when the volume of air breathed in is reduced the carbon dioxide in the lungs accumulates and this in turn will readjust the carbon dioxide threshold.

When asked for a simple definition of his theory, Professor Buteyko said it is this: the reduction of the depth of breathing by the relaxation of the respiratory muscles to create a little air shortage. Two words he directed at his patients were 'breathe less'. This is the very essence of Buteyko breathing.

Throughout this book each exercise and how it should be practised will be examined. However, it is important to always be aware of what is being achieved and why. Remember that overbreathing will trigger asthma and the intention is to learn to breathe a more correct volume by relaxation. Breathing can primarily be reduced by relaxing all the muscles involved in respiration. It is very important to relax the muscles because increased tension leads to overbreathing, reduces blood flow and therefore oxygenation.

A quote from sixth century BC philosopher Lao Tzu states: 'The perfect man breathes as if he does not breathe.' Through the Buteyko Method the individual learns to breathe in a calm, silent and still manner.

A diagram illustrating breathing patterns will accompany many of the exercises. The following symbols are used for each diagram. Refer to this diagram periodically in order to understand those that follow.

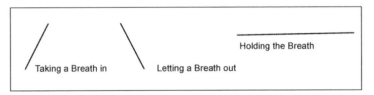

How to interpret breathing instructions

Nasal breathing. Why?

The nose has a number of features designed to bring cold dry outside air to a more acceptable condition before it enters the lungs. The mouth, however, is not intended to condition atmospheric air – it is merely for talking, eating and drinking.

Air that is drawn in through the nose passes along turbinates and spends a longer period of time in the body. This serves to warm the inhaled air far more effectively than drawing it in through the mouth.

Air is filtered by the turbinates and tiny hair-like structures that work to prevent pollen, dust and bacteria from entering the lungs. The sticky mucus blanket within the nose traps a significant proportion of all the bacteria and allergens contained in air. On any one day, a person with asthma may inhale from 10,000 to 20,000 litres of air laden with foreign particles including many triggers. Whereas the nose can remove these deposited particles within fifteen minutes, it takes 60–120 days for them to be removed from the small air sacs (alveolus) within the lungs.

Lungs require a warm moist environment and therefore it is imperative that the air drawn into the lungs meets this

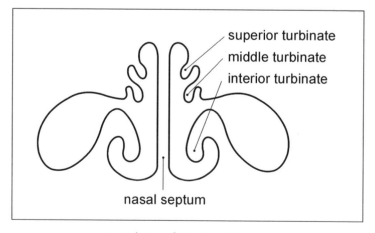

Frontal view of interior of the nose

condition. The nose humidifies inhaled air by increasing moisture content. A sign of good health is a moist nose while a dry nose can be a sign of dehydration. Take a moment now to think about a dog. Why a dog? Well, it's common knowledge that when Fido's nose is cool and moist, he's most likely to be healthy, but when his nose is dry and hot, his owner is probably facing a trip to the vet!

It is just as important to breathe out through the nose as it is to breathe in through it, despite a common conviction, particularly among sporting professionals, to the contrary. By breathing out through the nose, part of the moisture contained in the exhaled air is retained, thus reducing moisture loss. Breathing out through the mouth results in a greater loss of carbon dioxide and may lead to dehydration. This can be observed by breathing onto a pane of glass and then checking the residue of moisture left.

Nasal breathing helps to regulate volume. All mouth breathers overbreathe and as a result suffer some symptoms of hyperventilation. The nose is a smaller channel to breathe through, and therefore it helps to reduce the volume of air as there is about fifty per cent more resistance. It is possible to overbreathe through the nose but to a lesser extent.

Western research has concluded that the volume of air passing through the lungs of a person with asthma is usually between two and four times the norm.[1,2,3] From this it is possible to deduct that the quantity of allergens inhaled by a person with asthma is far greater than that of a person with healthy breathing. By switching to nasal breathing and reducing the volume of air taken in, the quantity of the allergens inhaled will be dramatically reduced, resulting in less exposure to triggers.

Some people will instinctively hold their breath whenever they come across a trigger, and this is a good idea. For example, if you are walking in the street and a bus emitting a large volume of fumes passes by, just breathe out, and try to hold your breath until you have walked away from the pollution. When you recommence breathing, reduce the volume so that the amount of polluted air entering the airways will be reduced.

A partially blocked nose is common with nasal breathing, one nostril will be partially blocked while the other is free to work. Check to see which of your nostrils is blocked by placing your finger over one nostril and breathing through the other; then repeat using the other nostril.

You will find that after three or four hours the blocked nostril will usually clear and the previously clear nostril will become blocked. This is a natural pattern which enables one nostril to rest at a time. During physical activity such as walking or light jogging, both nostrils will open up to allow more air into the body. When lying down at night, usually the lower nostril will be blocked and the upper nostril clear.

Mouth breathing results in irregular and erratic breathing while switching to nasal breathing brings more rhythm to the process.

The importance of breathing through the nose tends to receive very little attention from the medical profession. It seems to be accepted without question that some people will breathe through the mouth and others through the nose. However, breathing through the mouth is detrimental to your health and this is emphasised to all patients who learn breath retraining. Mouth breathers have generally poorer health and may go through life with an uncomfortable and permanently blocked nose. Furthermore, mouth breathers have a higher incidence of cavities and gum disease than those who breathe through their nose.[4]

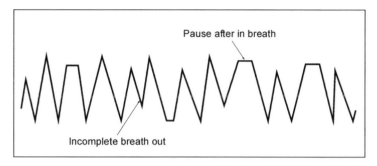

Erratic and irregular mouth breathing

It was observed by American artist George Catlin in the course of his nineteenth century travels in North America that the native Indian mothers paid a lot of attention to their infants' breathing. If at any time the baby opened its mouth to breathe, the mother would gently press the baby's lips together to ensure continued nasal breathing. George also noted that the rate of sickness and illness among the native Indian people was very low in comparison with European settlers.

'When I have seen a poor Indian woman in the wilderness, lowering her infant from the breast, and pressing its lips together as it falls asleep ... I have said to myself, "Glorious education! Such a mother deserves to be the nurse of Emperors". And when I have seen the careful, tender mothers in civilised life, covering the faces of their infants sleeping in overheated rooms, with their little mouths open and gasping for breath; and afterwards looked into the multitude, I have been struck with the evident evil and lasting

results of this incipient stage of education,' he wrote in his 'Notes of Travels Amongst the North American Indians' published in 1870.

It is vital to remember to breathe through the nose at all times and parents should also explain the importance of nasal breathing to their children. Parents will generally be the best judges of how to explain things but to help the child understand the importance of breathing through their nose, it might be helpful to explain to them the following way, using a little girl called Emily as our example:

The air that we breathe is not always clean. It can contain a large amount of dirt particles with germs, smoke and bacteria too small to be seen. The nose has tiny filters that clean this air before it goes into the body. If the air sneaks in through the mouth, we're sucking in dirty air. This is not good at the best of times but is particularly so if a child like you or an adult like me has an asthma problem.

Whenever the child sees or smells dirty air, get her to hold her breath and walk away from it. Explain that the less dirty air she breathes in, the less difficulty she will have with her asthma.

Air that sneaks in through the mouth is cold and dry and the body doesn't really like that. Air that comes in through the nose is warm and moist and is much better for the body. Ask Emily whether she would prefer to be warm (but not too warm) or very cold. She will hopefully answer that she prefers to be warm. Then explain that the body prefers warm air too but it can only get this nice warm air by breathing through the nose. If she tells you that she prefers to be cold then I'm afraid you're on your own explaining this one!

A note of caution

Now is the time to sound a note of caution. Before the Buteyko Clinic Method is commenced this section should be read carefully. While Buteyko Breathing is a perfectly safe therapy, it can involve an element of risk for people with particular illnesses or susceptibilities.

Please note the following in particular:

+ If you experience an exacerbation of your symptoms, then you are not doing the exercises correctly and you should stop until you establish that you can do them correctly.

  Do not commence breath retraining if you have any of the following conditions: sickle cell anaemia; arterial aneurysm; very high uncontrolled blood pressure; any heart problems in the past three months; uncontrolled hyperthyroidism; a known brain tumour or kidney disease.

+ If you suffer from any of the following, then you should only undertake breath retraining under the direct supervision of an experienced qualified Buteyko Clinic practitioner: diabetes; (a reversal of hyperventilation will reduce blood sugar levels which may in turn lead to a coma, exercises must be performed only with an experienced Buteyko practitioner in conjunction with an endocrinologist) severe asthma; emphysema; epilepsy; schizophrenia; unsatisfactory blood pressure levels or chest pains or pain in the heart region.

+ If you have any of the above conditions, or if you experience any distress, or are in any way unsure, please refrain from doing exercises involving holding the breath beyond the first feeling of a need for air. Exercises involving holding the breath include nose unblocking, maximum pause, breath-hold during physical exercise and *Steps*. If you are in any doubt as to whether breath retraining may be suitable for you, please contact an experienced qualified Buteyko practitioner.

What to expect

Roughly two thirds of those who apply breath retraining will experience a cleansing reaction within the first two weeks and each time the control pause increases by ten seconds. Reduced breathing leads to an increased blood flow and better oxygenation of all internal organs especially eliminatory organs. Cleansing reactions are indicative of the powerful physiological change which the body undergoes.

For people with asthma, the most common reaction is excess mucus from the nose and airways. For a few days and weeks, the nose may be runny, especially during physical activity with nasal breathing. It is also possible to experience an increased amount of mucus moving up from the lower airways. Mucus that was previously trapped is released by a dilation of the airways and is brushed upwards to the throat. If it is green or yellow, spit it out. Most importantly, do not force the mucus to the throat. If necessary a gentle throat clearing will suffice. Let the mucus come up naturally because forcing mucus up without addressing hyperventilation will only lead to the creation of more mucus.

In addition, you may experience other symptoms such as a slight headache, diarrhoea, nausea, excessive tiredness with increased yawning, mild depression, general flu like symptoms, insomnia, a bad taste from the mouth, foamy saliva, coloured urine, a greatly reduced appetite or a general feeling of being unwell. People who have been on a large course of steroids may be able to smell the tablets/medicine through their skin.

Do not be alarmed if you do experience some symptoms. This is simply your body readjusting to a healthier way of life. Symptoms are, in general, not disruptive and will pass in two or three days. Like any detoxifying process of the body, there is a short adjustment phase. Many people look forward to the reaction because it is direct feedback as their body cleanses itself after all those years of bad breathing.

Do the following to help reduce the intensity and duration of cleansing reactions:

+ Drink warm water regularly throughout the day.
+ Continue with reduced breathing by relaxation.
+ Take pain relievers, such as a headache tablet, if necessary.

Most importantly, do not stop doing the exercises when you experience a cleansing reaction. The symptoms are a direct result of overbreathing and the control pause (explained later) will increase when the cleansing reaction has passed.

On a positive note, everyone will experience signs of health improvement including: fewer asthma symptoms; less coughing, wheezing and congestion especially in the mornings; increased calmness and concentration; better sleep and more energy, and reduced appetite and cravings for coffee, chocolate and other foodstuffs.

Nose unblocking exercise

It was outlined earlier how a reduction in carbon dioxide levels causes an increase in mucus secretion and constriction of the airways. The nose forms part of the air system and is usually the first part to become constricted. The following is a simple exercise which will unblock the nose in as little as five minutes. It is based on temporarily increasing carbon dioxide levels in the blood, which will in turn open the nasal passages. This exercise is the same for both children and adults. At this point it is worth practising the exercise before you read further.

+ Sit upright on a straight-backed chair.
+ Normalise and calm your breathing. Take a small breath (two seconds) in through your nose, if possible, and a small breath out (three seconds). If you are unable to take a breath in through your nose, take a tiny breath in through the corner of your mouth.
+ Pinch your nose and hold your breath. Keep your mouth closed.
+ Gently nod your head or sway your body until you feel that you cannot hold your breath any longer. (Hold your nose until you feel a relatively strong need for air.)
+ When you need to breathe in, let go of your nose and breathe gently through it, in and out, with your mouth

closed. Avoid taking a deep breath when you breathe in, and calm your breathing as soon as possible by focusing on relaxation. Repeat to yourself 'relax and breathe less'.

✦ Continue to do this exercise until you can breathe through your nose fully. If your nose does not become totally unblocked, wait about two minutes and perform this exercise again. Initially you may need to do this a number of times before your nose is completely unblocked. This is yet another case of 'practice makes perfect'.

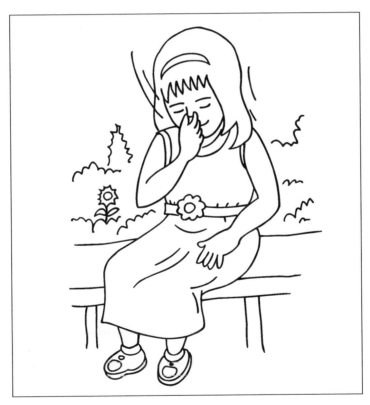

Unblocking the nose

After doing this exercise a few times your nose will be unblocked. If you continue to overbreathe, or take a deep breath, you will lose the additional carbon dioxide and your nose will become blocked again. Perform this exercise each time that your nose becomes blocked. Even if you have a cold, make sure to breathe through your nose. You may think you can't clear your nose when you have a heavy cold, but you can.

Holding the breath traps additional carbon dioxide which has been produced from the physical activity involved in moving the muscles. It is quite common for the nose to become blocked again shortly after doing this exercise. This is because the underlying breathing has not been changed and the body has not become accustomed to the increased carbon dioxide level. However, after some time, and with regular practice of breathing exercises, the body will adapt to a higher level of carbon dioxide and the nose will remain unblocked.

Warning call

Your nose is your first warning call – it is the first part of the airways to constrict if you are beginning to hyperventilate.

For example, much of my work involves presentations to groups of people: this can involve talking for up to four hours at a time. Frequently it happens that, towards the end of the four hours, I feel my nose becoming a little blocked. This is a direct result of the loss of carbon dioxide from excessive talking. My blocked nose is my indicator that I am breathing more than I should, so I take a break from talking and normalise my breathing.

Talking involves continuous air exhalation through the open mouth and the continuous loss of carbon dioxide. With a short period of reduced talking, or not talking, breathing will begin to normalise and the nose will unblock automatically.

Breathing too deeply through the nose will result in it becoming partially blocked. However it will not become fully blocked unless the switch is made to mouth breathing. This is because of the body's breathing defence mechanism. As soon as the nose becomes partially blocked, the volume of air is decreased; this causes the level of carbon dioxide to increase and in turn to dilate the nasal passages. Continuous overbreathing means the nose will become partially blocked once more which will again increase carbon dioxide. In turn, this will open the nasal passages and so on. It can feel a little uncomfortable trying to continue breathing through the nose as it starts to block. The best action to take therefore is to do the nose unblocking exercise or walk a number of steps holding your breath. This will quickly unblock the nose and make it feel comfortable again.

If you can hear yourself breathe through your nose (whistling) this is a warning that you are breathing too much. Breathing through the nose should be a silent activity.

When the switch is first made from mouth to nasal breathing, the volume of air being inhaled will reduce. The body may begin to play tricks and convince individuals to breathe more by inducing yawning, sighing, regular sniffing or the odd mouth breath. Try not to increase breathing at this point. When the need to deep breathe arises, for example during a sigh, swallow immediately. If the need to yawn also occurs, avoid taking the deep breath that accompanies a yawn. Instead stifle the yawn by keeping the mouth closed, or swallow.

It takes just a few days for a habitual mouth breather to change breathing to permanent nose breathing. Increasing observation of breathing, reducing volume of breathing and practising nose unblocking exercises are important elements in trying to make this change.

After the change to nasal breathing has been made, it will become uncomfortable to mouth breathe because the effects of cold dry air entering through the mouth will be felt. Often people begin to wonder how on earth they managed to go through life with a permanent, and very uncomfortable, blocked nose – a condition which is frequently, and usually unsuccessfully, addressed by the use of nasal sprays, decongestants or even an operation.

Nasal remedy

Those suffering constant nasal congestion and inflammation should practise nose unblocking exercises but also wash out the nose daily with the following remedy – especially those who have become dependent on nasal sprays.

Dissolve half a teaspoon of sea salt and half a teaspoon of bread soda (bicarbonate) in one pint of boiled water and let it cool. A plastic syringe with a rubber bulb can be purchased from a pharmacy. Fill this syringe with the solution and squeeze into one nostril while blocking the other nostril with a finger. Sniff the water in until it reaches the back of the throat. Spit it out and then repeat with the other nostril.

Another option is to cup the warm salt water into the hand and sniff the water up into the nose one nostril at a time (again with the other nostril blocked).

People who live near the sea find that sniffing up clean sea water is also effective. This is a traditional remedy which also works well for sinus problems.

Yogi have, for thousands of years, realised the benefits of nasal cleansing and use a special vessel called a neti pot to pour the solution into each nostril.

Pulse and control pause

Buteyko Clinic Method is a program of breath retraining aimed at reversing chronic hyperventilation on a permanent basis. While the exercises are very simple, it is important to follow them exactly as they are written in order to experience maximum benefits.

With breath retraining, there are two measurements that are used to monitor asthma severity and progress. These are the pulse, which is a measurement of the number of heart beats taken usually over a period of one minute, and the control pause [CP], which is the length of time for which you can comfortably hold your breath.

The peak flow meter will be a familiar piece of equip-
ment to many people with asthma. However it is not used as a measurement in Buteyko breathing. If peak flow

measurement is part of your asthma management, continue to use it. However, after taking a reading from your peak flow meter, hold your breath for three to five seconds and reduce your breathing for a while to replenish any loss of carbon dioxide.

Pulse

Everyone should be able to measure their pulse but it is especially important that asthmatics are able to do so. The pulse should be taken before and after each half-hour set of breathing exercises. When these exercises are performed correctly, with relaxation and reduced volume of breathing, the pulse at the end of exercise will be lower than at the start. Reducing breathing relaxes the smooth muscle of the arteries which results in less pumping work for the heart.

However, if breathing exercises are practised with too much effort or tension, the pulse will actually increase. It is important to spend time practising all breathing exercises with relaxation of muscles, even those involving physical activity.

It should also be noted that the pulse rate will vary throughout the day, depending on factors such as diet, eating patterns and activity levels.

As mentioned above, the pulse is measured by counting the number of heartbeats per minute. Another option is to measure the number of beats over thirty seconds and multiply by two. Measuring for fifteen seconds and multiplying by four leaves too much room for error and is not advisable.

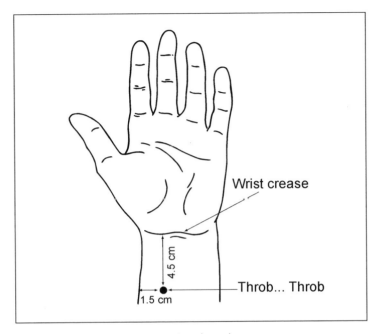

Wrist crease

4.5 cm

Throb... Throb

1.5 cm

Measuring the pulse

When measuring heartbeats, make sure to measure your pulse and not to count the number of seconds on your clock or watch.

Locate the pulse about one inch up from the wrist and about one centimetre inwards on the thumb side of the hand. Place two fingers from the free hand onto the groove or channel in this area of the wrist where the slight throb of the pulse can be felt through the fingertips.

If you have difficulty locating the pulse on the wrist then check for it at the carotid artery in the neck.

In general, the lower the resting heart rate, the healthier the individual is. Normal healthy adults will have a pulse rate of 60 to 80 beats per minute at rest. Physically fit individuals will have a lower pulse rate than this, although some individuals have a naturally low pulse rate.

If the pulse rate is greater than 90 and less than 110 beats per minute at rest, the asthma is uncontrolled and a visit to a doctor is necessary. If the pulse rate is greater than 110 beats per minute at rest, asthma is acute/severe and medical attention is necessary.

The normal pulse range for a child is higher than that of an adult. A child's pulse can vary from 60 to 100 beats per minute which decreases as the child gets older.

With both children and adults, an upward trend in the pulse or an increase of twenty per cent over 24 hours while taken at rest, are signs that asthma is deteriorating. Practising breathing exercises intensively will bring down the pulse and if necessary a doctor should be consulted to increase the dose of preventative medication.

It is advisable to note that the aforementioned pulse rate measurements must be only taken after resting for half-an-hour as the pulse rate increases considerably with physical activity.

The maximum recommended pulse rate for any individual while participating in physical activity is 220 minus their age. For example, the maximum recommended pulse rate for a twenty-five-year-old is 195 beats (220 minus 25) per minute.

The pulse will vary depending on a variety of factors. It may be adversely affected by, for example, food consumption levels, food allergies, stimulants such as coffee or chocolate, and factors such as excitement, anxiety, excessive talking and, of course, big breathing.

Control pause [CP]

The control pause is a measure of the level of carbon dioxide in the alveoli based on a comfortable breath hold. The control pause and pulse are used together to monitor asthma.

Over time, paying attention to the breathing pattern, your carbon dioxide threshold will adjust to a higher and healthier level. As a result the body becomes less sensitive to carbon dioxide accumulation, which will result in a gradual improvement in the length of time a person can hold their breath. By reducing the volume of breathing, carbon dioxide levels increase and therefore the control pause will increase.

Through overbreathing, the carbon dioxide level will decrease and therefore the control pause will decrease. The control pause will also decrease if medication is reduced too drastically.

The control pause is consistent and is a very good indicator of progress and of the current condition of the asthma, because of this it is essential to learn how to measure it correctly. Bear in mind that the control pause is only a measure; it is not an exercise to increase the level of your carbon dioxide.

The control pause enables the measurement of carbon dioxide in the alveoli without the need for any equipment other than a stopwatch or a watch/clock with a second hand.

Measuring your control pause

✦ Sit in an upright chair and adopt a good posture. Relax
  your shoulders and rest your lower back against the back
  of the chair.

✦ Do not change your breathing before taking your CP.
  Take a small breath in (two seconds) and a small breath
  out (three seconds). Hold your nose on the 'out' breath,
  with empty lungs but not too empty. Holding your nose is
  necessary to prevent air entering into the airways.

✦ Count how many seconds you can comfortably last before
  you need to breathe in again. Hold your breath until you
  feel the first need to breathe in. Release your nose and
  breathe in through it.

✦ Your first intake of breath after the CP should be no
  greater than your breath prior to taking measurement;
  you should not hold your breath for too long as this may
  cause you to take a big breath after measuring the CP.

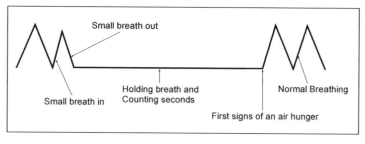

Measuring the Control Pause (a)

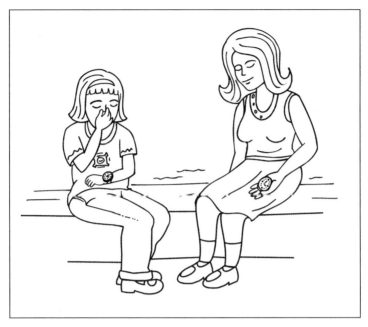

Measuring the Control Pause (b)

Points to bear in mind

There are a number of important points to bear in kind when measuring your CP. Breathe normally before taking your CP. Try not to take a big breath before you start as this will give an inconsistent reading.

If you have just completed breathing exercises, wait two or three minutes. Measuring your CP directly after exercises will give an inaccurate reading due to an existing air shortage from the exercise.

Do not breathe all the air out of your lungs because this will be very uncomfortable and will result in a reduced CP. Also do not try to hold your breath for too long as this will give an incorrect reading. The CP is a measurement of your progress only: it is not an exercise to see how long you can hold your breath before you burst!

Hold your breath only until you feel the first urge to breathe in. You may not like the result but it is the correct one and that's what you need to know. You can then take steps to correct it and gauge your progress with confidence.

It does take some practice before you become consistent in measuring your control pause. The measure is subjective because it is difficult to know what the first urge is. At first, it is very easy to push a little too hard and this is the case when the breath after taking the CP is greater than before.

With practice, the control pause will become more consistent. A reading of the level of carbon dioxide in the alveoli will be achieved with a correct control pause.

Carbon dioxide level

The level of carbon dioxide in the body determines the length of time the breath can be held: a higher level of carbon dioxide corresponds to a longer breath hold. The table above was developed by Professor Buteyko after he had measured the breath-holding ability of literally thousands of patients and matched it to their carbon dioxide levels. The figures are consistent and show the level of carbon dioxide based on the length of the control pause.

If the control pause is eight seconds, then there is a little less than four per cent carbon dioxide in the alveoli. If the control pause is fifteen seconds, the carbon dioxide is

	CO2 in alveoli [%]	Control pause [sec]
Perfect Health	6.5	60
	6.0	50
Asthma Free	5.5	40
	5.0	30
	4.5	20
	4.0	10
	3.5	5
	Death	

between four and four-and-a-half per cent. The aim is to increase the level of carbon dioxide to at least five-and-a-half per cent giving a control pause of forty seconds.

With continuous practice of exercises, the respiratory centre will become accustomed to a higher concentration of carbon dioxide. Remember, it is the level of carbon dioxide that determines the need to breathe.

Low control pause

A low control pause means the body's respiratory centre has become fixed at a low level of carbon dioxide and therefore will send instructions to breathe a large volume of air in order to maintain this level. By commencing breathing exercises, an attempt is made to break this pattern by deliberately reducing the volume of air inhaled.

Regular practice of exercises and increased observation of breathing will help the respiratory centre to become fixed at a higher level of carbon dioxide. Just as it took time for the respiratory centre to become accustomed to a low level of carbon dioxide, it will also take time for it to become accustomed to a new higher, and healthier, level.

The increase in CP is dependent on a variety of factors: the severity of the asthma, age, how much the breathing exercises have been practised and how much attention has been given to the breathing. The more attention to, and observation of, breathing the better.

The control pause is an accurate measure of the level of carbon dioxide in the alveoli. It therefore gives a very good indication of the state of a person's asthma and in fact, of health generally. If the control pause is increasing then the asthma is improving. If the control pause is decreasing the individual's asthma is getting worse.

A decreasing control pause is advance warning of an imminent attack. If the trend is for the control pause to decrease over a number of days, then it is important to take control of the condition by reducing the breathing to raise carbon dioxide levels. If it is not proving possible to increase the CP by breathing exercises, then it may be necessary to increase the level of preventative medication that has been prescribed.

A change in CP will often be noticed simply from observing reactions to various daily activities. It is possible to determine from the CP whether something is or is not good for asthma.

For example, if the CP has decreased following exercise, that person has been deep breathing during the exercise, so it would be important to change the way exercise is carried out. If the CP decreased following a large steak then eating large quantities of meat may not suit that individual or it may be that too much was eaten at one sitting. If the CP consistently drops at work then stress may be a factor or a reversal to mouth breathing may have occurred while concentrating on work. The CP gives excellent feedback and enables everyone to turn detective and determine whether something is a help or a hindrance to their asthma.

To determine whether breathing exercises are being practised correctly, it is necessary to measure the CP at the start of each exercise and several times during it to ensure that overbreathing is not occurring. The aim of breathing exercises is to reduce breathing volume, which will reset the carbon dioxide threshold and therefore the CP. The breathing exercises are being performed correctly when the CP increases a little between each set of exercises. Breathing exercises are being performed incorrectly when the CP is decreasing between each set. The pages towards the back of this book contain detailed exercise programs.

If it is proving impossible to influence the CP, then the exercises are not being done correctly and it would probably be better to stop doing the exercises and learn how to do them properly from an experienced practitioner.

From week to week, there should be a noticeable improvement in the control pause. The body will become conditioned to a higher level of carbon dioxide when breathing exercises are practised correctly. This will be reflected in a higher control pause. As far as Buteyko breathing is concerned, the control pause is the most important measurement of an individual's asthma.

Measuring the CP in the morning before breakfast gives the most important measurement of the state of a person's asthma. In the depths of sleep, breathing is a subconscious activity that cannot be interfered with. For this reason, the morning CP will give a true measurement of the level of carbon dioxide.

During the day, the CP will change depending on factors like eating, stress and talking, and on how the breathing changes. If the control pause is thirty seconds during the day and only ten seconds in the morning then the true control pause is ten seconds.

Peak flow meter

The peak flow meter, as used in conventional management, involves taking deep inhalations followed by large exhalations to measure the forced expiration of air in one second. This is an act of hyperventilation, and it can cause the airways to go into spasm, leading to inconsistent and inaccurate readings of the severity of asthma. In addition, blowing into a peak flow meter a number of times consecutively may be enough to start an attack. It is possible to continue to use your flow meter alongside the CP if desired. After taking a peak flow reading, the breath should be held for three to five seconds and the breathing reduced for three minutes to reverse the act of hyperventilation.

Scientists at Brunel University have recently devised a new product which allows people with asthma test their condition while they breathe normally. This device is based on capnography and measures the rate of change of carbon dioxide in exhaled air against time with normal breathing.

Measurements are reliable and simple to take allowing asthmatic patients to accurately monitor their condition. It is worth noting that this device recognises the importance of correct carbon dioxide levels. Overtime, it may help change the current understanding regarding the significance of carbon dioxide.

How severe is your asthma?

When most people with asthma commence Buteyko Clinic Method a control pause of between ten and twenty seconds will be experienced in between attacks. This means that they are habitually breathing enough air for five or six people.

If your morning control pause is less than ten seconds then you have a breathing volume greater than six times your body's requirements; you have a serious hyperventilation problem and your asthma is rated as severe.

If your morning control pause is 12 to 15 seconds then you are breathing five times the body's requirements, indicating you have chronic and nocturnal asthma.

If your morning control pause is 15 to 20 seconds you are breathing four times the body's requirements, indicating moderate asthma, nocturnal and exercise-induced asthma.

If your morning control pause is 20 to 30 seconds you are breathing three times the body's requirements, indicating that the main asthma symptoms have disappeared, although some nocturnal asthma persists.

If your morning control pause is 30 to 40 seconds you are breathing once-and-a-half times to twice the body's

requirements, indicating that you may have asthma symptoms after exposure to a severe trigger.

If your morning control pause is 40 to 60 seconds, then
your breathing is correct. As a direct result, your underlying
asthma is being treated and you will very rarely have symptoms.

If your morning control pause is sixty seconds you have
no health problems or diseases of civilisation. For over forty
years Professor Buteyko and his associates were unable to
find any person with a control pause of sixty seconds who
had any of the diseases of modern civilisation. Diseases of
civilisation are those which have become more widespread
as countries become more industrialised, including angina,
asthma, allergies, bronchitis, bronchiectasis, chronic fatigue
syndrome, diabetes, emphysema, hypertension, sleep apnoea
and many more.

chapter 3

taking control

"'Begin at the beginning," the king said gravely, "and go till you come
to the end; then stop.'"

— Lewis Carroll, *Alice's Adventures in Wonderland*

The overall aims of breathing exercises are to increase the
level of carbon dioxide in the alveoli, and to train the body to
become accustomed to it. As indicated in previous chapters,
our lungs require a concentration of between five per cent
and six-and-a-half per cent carbon dioxide, equating to a
control pause (CP), taken while at rest, of between forty and
sixty seconds. Most of those with an asthma problem will
have a CP of between 10 and 20 seconds, and this points to a
carbon dioxide level of between four and four-and-a-half per
cent. As you can see, this is much lower than what the body
requires.

To trap a higher level of carbon dioxide and to readjust
the respiratory centre to this increased amount, exercises
specifically aimed at reducing breathing are performed at
specific times each day. These exercises should be continued
until a reduced volume of breathing becomes a way of life,
and until the control pause reaches at least forty seconds.

When you are able to maintain a control pause of forty seconds, you will have mastered the art of correct breathing, it will be an unconscious activity, and will be incorporated into your daily life.

To increase the control pause to your interim target of twenty seconds, breathing exercises are essential. As you train yourself to breathe correctly, physical activity should be used in conjunction with breathing exercises to help increase the control pause from twenty to your ultimate aim of forty seconds.

The objectives of these exercises are:

+ To lower the incidence of asthma attacks.
+ To halt an attack at the first sign of symptoms. For example, a simple blocked nose is one of the first signs of an attack.

Over a twelve-month period, breathing is brought to the more normal level of three to five litres as shown in the following diagram. This breathing is best described as regular, calm and smooth.

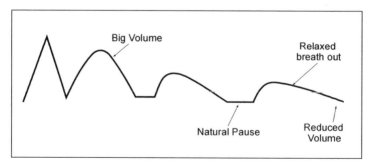

The change to correct breathing

The most important requirement before starting these exercises is to be aware of your breathing. If you are not aware of your breathing, you will not be able to reduce the volume of air drawn in and consequently you will not experience any improvement at all. I have included in this book a number of different breathing exercises. Choosing the most appropriate depends on a number of factors, such as whether you are an adult or a child, whether you have mild or severe asthma, whether you are having an attack or not, and whether or not you are physically exercising at the time.

As you read on, you will see that four breathing exercises are outlined in this chapter as follows:

Exercise One:	Reduced breathing by relaxation and monitoring air-flow with finger.
Exercise Two:	Reduced breathing for children.
Exercise Three:	Reduced breathing to overcome an asthma attack.
Exercise Four:	Reduced breathing during nose-blowing.

Exercise One

Reduced breathing by relaxation and monitoring air-flow with finger

The following is a very simplified version of one of the main exercises involved in breath correction. Certain steps have been omitted as it is essential they are practiced under the direct supervision of a practitioner to take into account individual nuances of the patient.

This exercise lasts about half-an-hour and it is recommended that you practice two to three times each day. If you can, you should practice before breakfast, during the day if possible, and again in the evening. Exercises should be carried out in a quiet place with no distractions. The temperature should be cool and the room airy because a hot and stuffy environment can promote big breathing, the exact opposite of what you are trying to achieve.

Food affects your breathing, so it is not recommended that you practice immediately after eating a meal. Exercises are best practised before meals or at least two hours after them. At half hourly intervals there should be pulse and control pause measurement, as well as a number of sets of breathing exercises.

If you want to get the best out of these exercises, it is recommended that you adhere to the following general guidelines. Go to a quiet place where you are unlikely to be disturbed and where you will have no distractions. Place a 'Do Not Disturb' sign on the door, if you need to, and take the telephone off the hook or switch off your mobile. You will need to concentrate to complete this exercise correctly, particularly in the early days.

Adopt a correct but comfortable posture. Correct posture involves sitting up straight with both feet underneath your chair. If you have difficulty with this, then imagine a thread suspended from the ceiling, attached to the top of your head, holding you in an upright position.

Correct posture is very important in helping to reduce your breathing. When you sit slouched, your breathing will

increase and will be more from the upper chest than the
tummy, where it should be coming from. When you adopt
the correct posture, your tummy will move more than your
upper chest and your breathing will require less effort. Your
tummy will move out with each inhalation (breathing in) and
will move in with each exhalation (breathing out) because of
the action of the diaphragm, which is the main breathing
muscle. Make sure that your tummy moves in the right
sequence. If not, you are performing what is known as
reverse breathing.

Now that you are in the right place and the right
posture for you, focus on your breathing. Feel the movement of air in and out of your body, particularly through
your nostrils. Concentrate on the slight movement your
body makes with each inhalation and exhalation. It is vital to
be aware of your breathing so that you can correct it. If you
are unaware of your breathing, you will not be able to
improve it.

As you breathe, let your shoulders fall to their natural
position. Raised or tense shoulders increase the volume of
the chest cavity and so increase the volume of air inhaled.
Tension increases breathing, but relaxation decreases it.
Relax the muscles involved in respiration, such as the
muscles above your tummy and in your chest.

The next step is to monitor the amount of air flowing
through your nostrils by placing your finger under your nose
in a horizontal position. Your finger should lie just above
your top lip, and close enough to your nostrils so that you
can feel the airflow, but not so close that the airflow is
blocked.

Now, breathe air slightly into the tip of your nostrils. Little breaths or short breaths mean the amount of air reaching your lungs reduces. By reducing the depth of your breathing or the length of each breath, in other words, the number of breaths you take every minute may increase, but don't worry because this is normal. Remember that the aim is to reduce the volume.

When you breathe out, the more warm air you feel, the bigger your breathing. Concentrate on reducing the amount of warm air you feel on your finger.

Don't worry if this exercise does not work for you the first time you try it. It will take time for your body to become accustomed to the lower volume of breathing. Over time it will become easier. A gradual and relaxed approach is best, because if you try to decrease the amount of air too quickly or too much, it may cause involuntary gasps of air or cause you to take bigger breaths. It is important that you get to the stage where you can sustain reduced breathing over the course of three to five minutes.

Take a few minutes' break before you start the next five minutes of reduced breathing. Two sets of twenty minutes

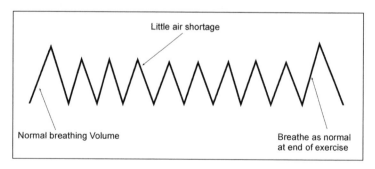

Creating a little air shortage

per day is the **minimum** time that should be spent on this exercise, combined with relaxation and observation of your breathing for the remainder of the day and night (more about this later). In order to make progress it is necessary to spend this amount of time practising. After a number of months, and depending on your progress, breathing exercises can be performed while doing any activity such as reading a book or watching television.

Correct Sequence

People with severe asthma should practice breathing exercises three times per day, preferably before breakfast, before lunch and in the evening. For those with mild and moderate asthma, breathing exercises should be practised twice daily, before breakfast and before going to bed. For correct exercise practice, each block should take about half-an-hour to do correctly.

A block of exercises consists of:

1. Take your pulse, and note it.
2. Control pause.
3. Reduced breathing for five minutes.
4. Control pause.
5. Reduced breathing for five minutes.
6. Control pause.
7. Reduced breathing for five minutes.
8. Control pause.
9. Reduced breathing for five minutes.

10. Control pause.

11. Check your pulse again and compare with your pulse rate when you started the exercise.

In order to reset the respiratory centre you must spend at least fifteen minutes doing breathing exercises. The control pauses **in between** each set of breathing exercises may decrease due to accumulation of carbon dioxide. It is vital that the pulse at the end of exercise (11) has decreased and the control pause (10) has increased due to a readjustment of the respiratory centre to a higher level of carbon dioxide. If your results are different, it means that you are overbreathing during the exercises, but this can be corrected by applying greater relaxation and reducing the intensity of the air shortage created.

I am very familiar with what happens when the exercises are not done correctly. When I first started using the Buteyko method myself, I tried to reduce the depth of my breathing by tensing my stomach to influence the amount of air I inhaled. However, this led to an increase in my breathing because of the additional tension I created. When I learned how to do the exercise correctly, I then had to begin reversing my previous breathing pattern.

Your lower respiratory muscles can become tense in response to a decreased volume of breathing, so the best advice is to try to relax throughout the exercises. Some will find this more difficult than others – some people are, by nature, more relaxed than others – but relaxation is a priority.

Summary of Exercise One

+ Set aside time when you will have no distractions.
+ Sit down and adopt the correct posture.
+ Relax your respiratory muscles.
+ Place your finger under your nose without blocking the air-flow.
+ Concentrate on reducing the amount of air that is blown onto your finger by monitoring the temperature of the air you are breathing out through your nose.
+ Reduce volume by taking very small breaths.
+ Your control pause should increase when the exercises have been completed.
+ Your pulse should decrease when the exercises have been completed.

Exercise Two

Reduced breathing for children

We use a different method, called 'Steps', to help children understand the process of improving their carbon dioxide levels, simply because children may have difficulty using Exercise One. More detailed information on helping children is contained in Chapter Nine.

Steps is also helpful as a measurement of progress, particularly if the child has difficulty in applying the control pause correctly. Steps involves moving the muscles to increase the carbon dioxide level, and this is then

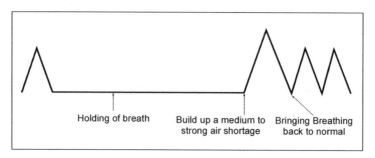

Doing *Steps*

combined with the child holding the breath, which will help to retain it.

For the purposes explaining this exercise, let's imagine again that you're dealing with a child called Emily. To perform *Steps* Emily should:

✦ Take a small breath in for two seconds and a small breath out lasting three seconds.

✦ Hold her breath by pinching her nose. It's better if Emily holds her nose by raising her hand above her mouth so that her mouth is visible. This way, if she takes a breath in through her mouth, it will be noticed.

✦ Get her to walk as many steps as she can until she needs to breathe in again. During *Steps*, encourage Emily to build up a large air shortage by doing as many steps as she can manage before she breathes in. Ensure she doesn't overdo it. If she does, it could become too stressful for her, and could put her off the exercises altogether.

✦ Encourage Emily to walk as many steps as possible, count aloud every five or ten steps, again ensuring that she doesn't overdo it.

✦ When Emily starts breathing, it must be only through her nose and her breathing must be calmed immediately. If her shoulders rise or become tense, point this out to her, and ask her to let her shoulders drop to the normal resting position.

✦ After completing *Steps* the first breath will usually be bigger than normal. Make sure Emily reduces or suppresses the second and third breaths.

✦ Get her to relax, by explaining that a relaxed body is like jelly on a plate, so that there is no tension and the muscles go all floppy. The more Emily relaxes, the quicker will be her recovery of normal breathing.

✦ Count each step aloud and record the number. Compare each day's steps with the previous day's so that progress can be measured.

Measurement tool

If a child is unable to do the control pause correctly, the *Steps* exercise – the best way of increasing carbon dioxide levels – can be used as a measurement tool. Always encourage the child to increase their steps over time. The goal is for the child to be able to walk a hundred paces without having to take a breath. *Steps* should be done only while walking. Reasonably fast walking is fine, but the child should not run.

If the child feels a relatively strong need to inhale following completion of *Steps*, then the exercises are being done correctly. If the child seems to be getting stressed just get her to reduce the number of steps she is taking so that it is not stressful for her.

Make sure to calm the deep breath sometimes taken on completion of the exercise. The *Steps* exercise is interspersed with reduced breathing called 'mouse breathing' and details are contained in the special chapter for children.

Two to three sets of *Steps* should be practised each day, depending on the severity of the asthma condition, and the more severe the condition the greater the number of sets should be completed each day. If the child has severe asthma however, then do make sure that she doesn't overdo it. Mind you, this applies equally to adults! Don't push a child too hard. Breathing exercises are not meant to be stressful, because increased stress is completely counter-productive; it will cause increased breathing, and the child may not be willing to continue with the exercises.

Again, the best times for the *Steps* exercises are before breakfast in the morning and at night, just before going to bed.

Correct sequence for children

CP	Steps	Steps	Steps	CP	Steps	Steps	Steps	mouse breathing	CP

Rest for about one minute between each set of *Steps*.

Exercise Three

Reduced breathing to overcome an asthma attack

An asthma attack involves faster breathing and bigger breaths than normal. When you have an attack, your respiratory centre is excited and you experience a very strong feeling that you simply cannot get enough air, so you are stimulated into trying to take bigger breaths, each with more volume than you would normally inhale. When an attack strikes, starting this exercise will be totally contrary to what you will feel like doing because it involves reducing your air intake even though you will feel an overwhelming urge to inhale as deeply as you can.

Throughout my teenage years my first instinct when the first signs of symptoms appeared was to reach into my pocket for my Ventolin reliever. What I know now is that this instinctive reaction creates a dependency on the drug, and a psychological addiction to it. Practice this exercise for the first few minutes to try to get over the attack before taking your reliever if your symptoms are mild enough. Of course, if the attack is severe, you must take your inhaler straight away.

+ First, sit down in an upright position. If you happen to be lying down in bed when the symptoms first appear, then get out of bed and sit down comfortably. If the room is stuffy, open the window to let in some fresh air.
+ At the first signs of an attack resist the urge to take big breaths, and focus on trying to reduce your breathing. It

may help if you repeat these words in your head, over and over: 'relax and remain calm'.

✦ When you decrease your breathing, be careful not to decrease it too much that you start to gasp.

✦ If you do create a strong need for air, be careful not to exacerbate your attack by taking in very big breaths afterwards.

With all asthma attacks, senses of panic, urgency and irritability can set in quickly, but these are the normal human responses generated when you feel a threat of suffocation. Always remember that **your attack is caused by your over-breathing** and try to remain as relaxed as you can during the attack. Clear your mind by focusing on your breathing as much as you can and practice the exercise above. You may not always stop an asthma attack using this exercise, but you can certainly reduce it substantially. Over time, as your condition improves, your ability to stop an attack will also improve.

If your attack lasts more than five minutes, take your reliever medication. If you are having a severe attack, then take medication immediately. If you are not responding to medication within ten minutes, seek medical attention immediately.

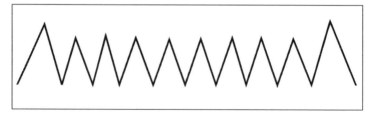

Reduced breathing during an asthma attack

If your symptoms are manageable, then try to overcome the attack by practicing the exercise for the first couple of minutes. If you are unable to obtain relief after five minutes, take your reliever medication. Do not prolong the attack or experience unnecessary discomfort by delaying the taking of the reliever unnecessarily. After you have taken your reliever medication, continue to remain relaxed and reduce your breathing.

The aim of this therapy is to reduce the number of attacks arising in the first place. While you will continue to experience attacks, the frequency will diminish as your control pause gets closer to the forty-second target.

Breathing exercises will only alleviate asthma when applied during the early stages of an attack or wheezing. If an asthma attack has been occurring for more than five minutes, it will be a lot more difficult to control using breathing exercises, especially if your normal control pause is less than twenty seconds.

It is very important that everyone with an asthma condition **continues to take their preventer treatment as prescribed** and has reliever medication at hand in case it's needed.

Exercise Four

Reduced breathing when blowing your nose

Slight colds contribute to asthma symptoms. Every time you blow your nose, some carbon dioxide is lost. Blowing your nose too much will result in an excessive loss of carbon dioxide. This will lead to an increase in the production of mucus, and you will then blow your nose to clear the mucus, resulting in a further loss of carbon dioxide, which will in turn create more mucus. Blowing the nose can be the catalyst for a vicious circle of nose clearing, carbon dioxide loss and mucus creation.

+ Try not to blow your nose but, if you must, do so only when absolutely necessary.
+ Blow your nose gently. Blowing your nose forcibly causes a greater loss of carbon dioxide and can also exacerbate sinus or ear problems.
+ After blowing your nose, hold your breath for a period equal to roughly half the length of your control pause.
+ Reduce your breathing.
+ For a child, do a set of *Steps* as outlined in Exercise Two in this chapter.

chapter 4

make correct breathing a habit

'The beginning of a habit is like an invisible thread, but every time we repeat the act we strengthen the strand, add to it another filament, until it becomes a great cable and binds us irrevocably, thought and act.'

— Orison Swett Marden

Physical exercise, talking, laughing and even sleeping influence our breathing patterns. In fact, everyday activities all have a role to play in the way we breathe so therefore it is necessary that we reduce the possibility of hyperventilation during them.

This chapter is sub-divided into:

Exercise Five: Reduced breathing while speaking or laughing.

Exercise Six: Reduced breathing while sleeping.

The breathing muscles.

Exercise Seven: A strategy for abdominal breathing.

Other breathing exercises.

Exercise Five

Correct breathing while speaking or laughing

For people with asthma, speaking for long periods of time can trigger symptoms. Frequently at workshops people remark: 'my coughing really starts at a meeting, or when I speak for long periods.' There is a direct relationship between a person's asthma problems and the amount of time spent talking, therefore this may help to explain why teachers make up the single largest professional group attending our workshops.

In a classroom environment, particularly if it's overheated or stuffy, recurrent chest infections and exacerbation of an asthma condition are common complaints. Indeed classrooms can contribute to the spread of colds and flu and it is likely that teachers are particularly susceptible due to the amount of talking they routinely do: excessive talking can weaken the immune system from excessive loss of carbon dioxide.

Here are some suggestions which may help in addressing this problem:

✦ Be aware of the need to minimise the amount of talking you do. Teachers or lecturers can use other means of communication such as video, tapes, CDs or even internet sourced items. Students could be encouraged to contribute more by reading or discussions. This can also be an effective way to generate interest and debate.

✦ Try not to take a deep breath in through your mouth prior to talking. This will be difficult initially as because you concentrate on what you are going to say, so trying to pay attention to your breathing at the same time will not come easily or naturally. Practice talking in front of a mirror for a few minutes each day, saying anything you like (the alphabet for example). If you are unable to breathe through your nose prior to every sentence, then start with just your first sentence and get that right. Then try for two sentences, then three and so on.

✦ Newsreaders use a particular style to add drama to their stories and many people unconsciously try to adopt this approach. This involves taking large breaths prior to long sentences in higher pitched tones. Many of the more severe hyperventilators I have met fit this pattern. Their sentences are unusually long and interspersed with deep upper chest breathing. The aim is to relax your speech, slow it down and reduce the emotional intensity of it.

✦ Long sentences result in a large exhalation of carbon dioxide, so aim to shorten your sentences. This will add a sense of calm to what you are saying, and you will be more easily understood. Natural mid-sentence pauses are good.

✦ An asthma sufferer can be easily identified in a telephone conversation because they inhale noisily, deeply and often with a wheeze, through the mouth before speaking. Aim to ensure that your breathing is quiet while you are talking because noisy breathing is indicative of over-breathing. Adopting nasal breathing and becoming more aware of your breathing during talking will help to reduce hyperventilation.

✦ Observe how other people breathe while they speak. This will help you with your own breathing techniques. Look out for sharp inhalations of air and movement of the upper chest while others talk.

✦ As you become more competent and relaxed at breathing through your nose while you speak, try talking at the end of an exhalation rather than directly after an inhalation. This will further conserve carbon dioxide during speech. For example:

Gently breathe in

Gently <..................> breathe <..................> out

Towards the end of your gentle out-breath, start talking. After the first comma in your sentence, take a gentle breath in and let a gentle breath out. Start talking again.

Laughter is the best medicine

Laughter has been described as the best medicine for many ills, but you must learn to control your breathing during it. Constant laughter involves deep inhalations and exhalations causing a loss of carbon dioxide. A number of experts have recognised the role of laughter in contributing to asthma symptoms.[1,2]

During laughter, try to:

✦ Reduce fits of laughter.

✦ Laugh with your mouth closed.

✦ Breathe in only through your nose.

✦ Hold your breath afterwards for a few seconds to replenish any loss of carbon dioxide.

Sometimes you just have to give way to a fit of laughter; you can't help it. But do help yourself to get your breath back by reducing your breathing.

Exercise Six

Correct breathing during sleeping

Many patients tell me that their symptoms are worse during the night or first thing in the morning. Some even say that it takes them hours every morning to get their breathing right. Symptoms such as a blocked nose, excessive mucus, tiredness, chest tightness, wheezing and breathlessness are common. These problems are usually caused by incorrect breathing while sleeping, and it is for this reason that we need to pay particular attention to how we breathe when we are asleep.

The risk of an asthma attack is greatest during sleep. Statistics show that most attacks occur between the hours of 3.00 and 5.00 a.m. Professor Buteyko's theory is that the natural position for humans is upright because when we lie down, our breathing increases automatically in comparison with the needs of our metabolism. For someone who is already overbreathing, this further increase in breathing will lead to a further depletion of carbon dioxide levels, and this can in turn lead to an attack.

Oversleeping is not good either. A good rule of thumb is to sleep only when you feel tired. This is when your body is telling you that sleep is necessary and generally seven to eight hours per night is enough. If you feel the need to sleep during the day, take a nap for twenty minutes while sitting upright. Correct breathing will increase your energy level and reduce fatigue so additional sleep should not be necessary. As your CP increases, the number of hours sleep you need each night should gradually decrease – probably to somewhere between five or six.

Reduced breathing during the day will help to reduce overbreathing at night, but we have very little control of our breathing in the depths of our slumbers. Because of this, there are a number of recommendations that may be followed to help ensure correct breathing at night.

Sleeping positions

Sleeping on your back is generally the worst position for someone with asthma. Your lower jaw drops and mouth breathing is almost inevitable. In this position, there is very little restriction to breathing and so breathing becomes deeper. Snoring, which is also caused by overbreathing and breathing through the mouth, is worse while sleeping on your back.

Increased blood pressure and bad health are just some of the side effects of snoring, not to mention the strain it can put on even the most harmonious of marriages. (I was in a youth hostel one night many years ago where a severe snorer was in danger of suffering grievous bodily harm from the adjoining bunk – and the general consensus was that he would have deserved it!) Another condition which affects children especially is bed wetting. For years Buteyko advocated that bed wetting was caused by hyperventilation. Now new research, published in *New Scientist*, confirms his view: 'Breathing problems are to blame for many cases of bedwetting in children, and perhaps in some adults too. And a simple treatment might solve the problem within weeks.'[3]

Changing from sleeping on your back to sleeping on your side may take some time. It may be helpful to place a number of pillows behind you while you sleep on your side. Another suggestion would be to wear a rucksack on your back filled with clothes or a football, and then there is the old wives' tale of sewing a tennis or golf ball into the back of your nightwear. All of these options may sound a little eccentric,

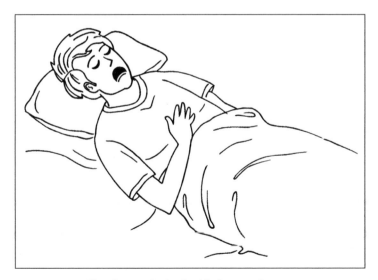

Sleeping on the back with the mouth open

but they will reduce the likelihood of you rolling onto your back and you should, over time, switch to sleeping on your side or tummy.

After years of research, Professor Buteyko came to the conclusion that people who sleep on their left side, in the foetal position, tend to breathe less deeply. The reason for this is thought to be variation in lung capacity: the lung which is closest to the bed performs most of the work and, as the left lung is smaller than the right, the volume of air brought through the lungs is reduced. Some people address the problem by sleeping with four or five pillows under the head. This has the effect of raising the head and chest above the level of the rest of the body, and a little nearer to a vertical position. A hard mattress, which restricts frontal movement of the body, can also help to reduce breathing. A soft mattress, particularly something like a water bed, is not good for correct breathing because it offers too little resistance.

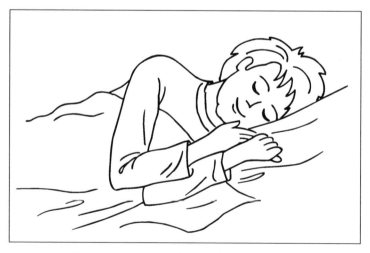

Sleeping on the left side with the mouth closed

Never eat before sleep

Eating a meal or drinking a protein-rich drink such as milk or hot chocolate two or even three hours before going to bed will result in increased breathing. Then you will have both an increase in breathing due to lying in a horizontal position, and an increase in breathing due to eating or drinking. Then overbreathing is guaranteed, resulting in a poor night's sleep. Eating a meal late at night can also result in having no appetite for breakfast.

Eating late at night on a regular basis is inherently unhealthy for anyone – asthmatic or not. It contributes to increased weight gain and lethargy, and it can disrupt the appetite the following day. My grandfather was a man of much wisdom and he had a saying that you should 'always wake up with an appetite'. I'm sure he was right.

Breathing through the nose at night

While sleeping it is important to breathe only through your nose. Mouth breathing will reverse the benefits of reduced breathing during the day. If you neglect your breathing for seven or eight hours every night then it will be impossible to change your breathing pattern on a permanent basis.

Here are some suggestions which will help you make a permanent switch to nasal breathing while sleeping:

✦ The guardian angel

One suggestion which may be suitable for children, is to have someone watch over you until you become more used to breathing through your nose at night. The role of this person is to close your mouth gently when you begin to mouth breathe, or to wake you if your breathing becomes too deep. A confirmed insomniac might fill the bill; otherwise, good luck in your search for a guardian angel!

✦ The hat or scarf

For children get a hat with a strap that comes under the chin. Cut most of the material from the hat so that there is just enough to keep the structure intact. Cutting away as much material as possible prevents the child from becoming too warm during the night because this would contribute to overbreathing. Get the child to wear the hat to bed and bring the strap under the chin to stop the lower jaw dropping down. A variation on this theme is to wrap a scarf around the child's head and under the chin. Tie it to ensure that the lower jaw is unable to drop down during the night. Both of these suggestions could be consigned to the 'off the wall' category by image-conscious children. However, with these suggestions in mind Asthma Care is currently in the process of having a special type of headwear designed to allow nighttime nasal breathing with minimum discomfort.

✦ Paper tape

From my experience, this is the idea that works best. Taping was first suggested by Buteyko's patients and has been used successfully by thousands of people in Russia, Australia, New

Zealand and the UK. If you feel that the tape is not for you, then use any of the above options (or one of your own) to prevent mouth breathing during the night. I have been using this option on and off for a number of years now, and I find it very beneficial if, for any reason, I am having any difficulty breathing through my nose at night.

The idea is to tape over the mouth with some sort of sticky paper. Make sure your mouth is completely closed before applying the tape. If your mouth is partially open, then you will be able to breathe through the tape during the night. I have found that the most suitable tape is 1 inch Medilite paper tape. Apply it horizontally to cover the mouth. If you are unable to place it in a horizontal position, then place it verti-cally. Before placing, remove much of the glue on it by sticking the tape to your hand and peeling it off a number of times. Do this until there is just enough glue to hold the tape in place. Before placing the tape on your mouth, make two tabs by putting a small fold at two of the corners. This will ease the task of removing the tape in the morning. The tape should not to be used on a child less than five years of age, and any child using it must be able to remove the tape during the night if they feel they need to. The tape should not be used if you are feeling nauseous or if you have been drinking alcohol.

If you are having difficulty breathing during the night while using the tape, then do reduced breathing exercises. Try not to remove the tape as, if you do, you are likely to begin to mouth breathe during your sleep and this will only make your symptoms worse.

It is possible that some people may, very reasonably, experience a feeling of panic at the very thought of having their mouth taped. To help overcome this it may be helpful to put the tape on half an hour before going to bed. This should be enough time to become used to the tape and to overcome any nervousness. For the first few nights wearing the tape will feel a little strange. It may come off during the night, but at least you will have spent some hours breathing through your nose. Continue to wear the tape until you have managed to change to breathing through your nose at night. How long this takes will vary with the individual.

If your nose is partially blocked before going to bed, then first clear your nose by completing the nose unblocking exercise outlined earlier. While wearing the tape, your nose will never completely block. If you are breathing deeply during the night while wearing the tape, your nose will partially block. This is the body's defence mechanism to prevent over breathing. However, when the nose becomes partially blocked, the level of carbon dioxide in the body will increase and this will unblock the nose. If you continue to overbreathe, your nose will become partially blocked again which will increase the level of carbon dioxide thus causing the nose to unblock and so on. Remember, your nose will only block completely if you switch to mouth breathing.

Reminder

Do not use the tape on a child if the child is unable to remove it easily themselves, or is unhappy about it. Do not use the tape if you are feeling nauseous, or have been doing any serious drinking.

Indicators of mouth breathing whilst sleeping

You will know you are mouth breathing if:

+ You wake up during the night breathing through your mouth, or
+ Your mouth is dry in the morning.

Having a wet mouth in the morning does not always indicate nasal breathing at night. Your mouth may close towards the end of your sleep and you will not be aware of your breathing prior to this. If you have a tendency to mouth breathe during the night, it is important to check for this dryness every morning. Your partner, or room mate, may also be able to tell you if you have been mouth breathing. They will certainly have no hesitation telling you if you have been snoring!

The last word on this topic

Some of the solutions outlined above may seem a bit extreme. However, most of them will only be needed until you get your asthma problem under control. At that stage, when your CP is consistently above 40 as a matter of course, you should find that your breathing while you sleep will be normal (and nasal) and no special measures will be necessary. The extreme remedies are suggested in order to help you to reach that stage.

Summary of correct sleeping

+ Be aware of any symptoms.
+ Try to sleep on your left side.
+ Never eat late at night. Don't be afraid to go to bed hungry; it won't do you any harm.
+ Breathe only through the nose at night.
+ Monitor your night breathing by checking your CP first thing in the morning.

Our breathing muscles

The three main groups of muscles used for breathing are the diaphragm, intercostal and accessory. Adopting diaphragmatic breathing is important for reducing hyperventilation.

The diaphragm is a strong, thin, flat sheet of muscle which separates the chest from the tummy and is shaped like the dome of an umbrella. To breathe in, the Medulla Oblongata, located in the brain, sends a message to the diaphragm to move downwards. This creates a negative pressure in the chest cavity, called the thorax, which causes the lungs to draw in air to equalise this negative pressure. The downward movement of the diaphragm on the abdominal contents causes the stomach to expand a little as we breathe in.

Two activities which result in poor use of the diaphragm are bad posture and mouth breathing. Mouth breathers tend to breathe using their upper chest muscles. Surprisingly, the upper chest does not expand outwards but rises and falls with each inhalation and exhalation. Switching to nasal

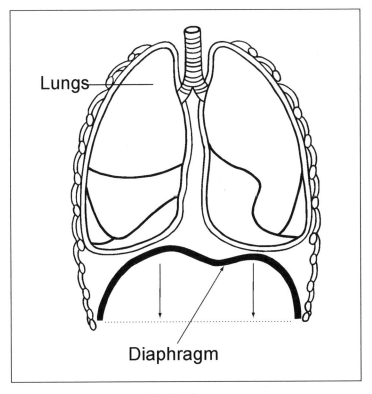

Lungs

Diaphragm

The Diaphragm

breathing is the first step in changing to diaphragmatic breathing.

Poor posture has a negative impact on breathing and being slouched over a desk all day will not help. At each workshop, I demonstrate how posture influences breathing.

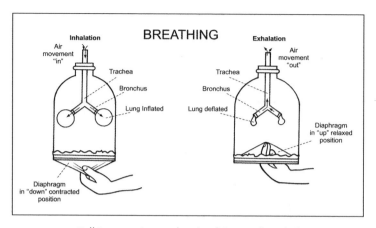

Bell Jar experiment showing 'How we breathe'

Note: *This bell jar experiment illustrates the central role which the diaphragm performs during breathing. To breathe in, neurons within the brain stimulate the diaphragm to contract (move downwards 1 cm to 10 cm) which enlarges the chest cavity or thorax. This causes a negative pressure (as in the first diagram) resulting in inhalation – until the pressure in the alveoli within the lungs equals atmospheric pressure. At the end of inspiration, the nerves to the diaphragm cease firing and so the muscles involved in respiration relax. This 'compresses' the air within the alveoli, and this causes an exhalation. It is the movement of the diaphragm from the relaxed position to the contracted position which causes the tummy to move out, and that from the contracted position to the relaxed position which causes the tummy to move in.*

'Deep' versus 'big'

The correct interpretation of the word 'deep' in this context is breathing using the diaphragm. A deep breath means using the depth of the lungs. There is a misconception that a deep breath is a big breath. A deep breath can be a big or a small breath. What is important is that the diaphragm moves. From time to time, I ask people to take a deep breath and the response is almost always huge inhalations of air – often through the mouth. Not only is this breathing big, it is also shallow as chest muscles predominate and only the top parts of the lungs are ventilated.

Exercise Seven

Strategy for abdominal breathing

'As we free our breath (through diaphragmatic breathing) we relax our emotions and let go our body tensions.'

— Gay Hendricks

To find out if you are breathing with your diaphragm:

✦ Hold one hand across your breastbone and the other hand on your tummy. At rest there should be no upper chest movement and only very small movement of the tummy. The tummy will expand as you breathe in and contract as you breathe out. For this exercise, do not wear

a very tight fitting belt, or clothes that will restrict abdominal breathing. It may help if you open the top button of
your trousers if it is unduly restrictive.

✦ Sit up straight and adopt a correct posture.

✦ Imagine that the back of your head is lightly suspended
by a thread from the ceiling.

✦ Lengthen the distance from your sternum (chest bone) to
your navel.

✦ Have both feet flat on the floor.

✦ Relax your shoulders and upper chest; this is very important.

✦ With your lips lightly together, breathe in gently through
your nose.

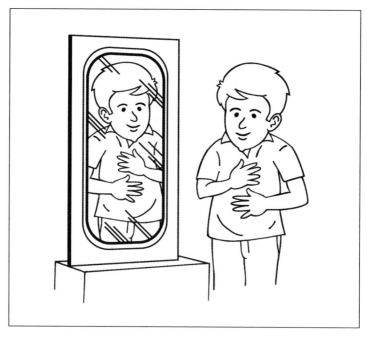

Seeing what part of the body moves the most

+ Place one hand on your chest and one hand on your tummy.
+ Concentrate on having very little movement of the upper chest.
+ Gradually reduce the amount of movement in your chest; having your hand on your chest will register this.
+ With your other hand, direct your attention to feeling your tummy move out with each inhalation and in on each exhalation.
+ Repeat to yourself: breathe out – tummy in; breathe in – tummy out.

OUT – IN

IN – OUT

+ Imagine a loose elastic band around your waist stretching slightly (but only slightly) as you inhale, and contracting as you exhale.
+ Focus on your stomach expanding with each inhalation and contracting with each exhalation. These movements are noticeable but slight.

Practice this for ten minutes each day, in addition to your exercises, until you have reduced upper chest breathing considerably. It is important not to practice for more than ten minutes at a time because breathing muscles can become very tired.

Remember

Breathe in – tummy out

Breathe out – tummy in

Other breathing exercises

There are many and varied breathing therapies, plenty of which I have tried, particularly when I was really suffering from my asthma. However, I can honestly say that Buteyko is the only one that has ever produced lasting results for me. There is evidence to support the credibility of Buteyko. From scientific trials and reported verbal evidence to the testimonials of literally thousands of people worldwide, no breathing therapy has matched the results of a proper application of the Buteyko Method. Indeed none has achieved the demonstrable and permanent success levels that Buteyko has achieved.

Some breathing exercises consist of blowing air as hard as you can through a straw to move marbles or blowing up balloons in order to increase lung capacity. Other exercises involve taking very big deep breaths in through the nose and out through the mouth. These are all taught with good intentions, but they are, in my opinion, likely to exacerbate your asthma rather than help it.

Forceful exhaling causes too much carbon dioxide to be carried out with each breath. A forced breath out results in the subsequent inhalation being large. This loss of carbon dioxide will cause spasm of smooth muscle, increased mucus and can lead to an asthma attack. An estimated 80 per cent of asthma sufferers will experience an attack from big breathing within two minutes. It is logical therefore to conclude that breathing exercises involving big breathing will produce the same symptoms in a relatively short period of time. Instead of increasing lung capacity, these exercises will lead to increased mucus and spasms causing airway obstruction.

Another misguided practice involves the forceful removal of mucus with coughing exercises or tapping of the back. Mucus is part of the body's defence mechanism against loss of carbon dioxide. Forcibly removing mucus results in increased breathing causing a loss of carbon dioxide. This will create more mucus. To remove mucus, practice reduced breathing exercises as outlined earlier. In addition, one could drink a glass of warm water with a $\frac{1}{4}$ teaspoon of sea salt dissolved in it, although some people find this too severe.

The mucus will be released as the airways open and will be brushed upwards to the pharynx by cilia, which are fine hair-like structures lining our airways. The mucus can then be harmlessly swallowed. If the mucus is green or yellow, it may be infected so it is better to spit it out. Note that yellow or green mucus is not always indicative of an infection. Mucus can be coloured by the presence of a large concentration of cells involved in inflammation such as eosinophils. Unfortunately, this may be interpreted as an infection and so antibiotics will be prescribed.[4] The overuse of antibiotics produces multi resistant strains of bacteria resulting in common infections not responding to antibiotic treatment at all.[5]

By reducing breathing, the body has no need to create additional mucus as part of its defence mechanism, and mucus already created will be removed naturally by airway dilation.

During the first couple of weeks of breath retraining, you will notice a considerable movement of mucus from the lower airways. This is part of the cleansing reaction.

Yoga

Many people ask about the role of yoga in addressing asthma problems. Yoga involves body posture and controlled breathing with deep breaths, and pauses which are effectively breath holds. People in the East would spend a large part of their day meditating in isolation, with no talking and on restricted diets, which would result in increased CO_2. Having spent many years practising, a yogi may have a control pause of as much as 180 seconds. For those with asthma the therapeutic benefits derived from yoga are a result of the reduced volume of breathing. While the inhalation is deeper, the number of breaths per minute may be as low as one or two. When practised correctly, breathing volume will reduce, sometimes dramatically.

My view is that, unless there is reduced breathing, there is very little therapeutic value to be gained for an asthmatic, although the relaxation will in itself reduce breathing and this is beneficial. If you are practising yoga, do not breathe in through your nose and out through your mouth as it will cause big breathing and dehydration.

A practice of some Eastern yogi is to seal both of their nostrils with beeswax in which is embedded a horse hair. They remove the horse hair leaving a tiny hole through which they breathe. As the volume of air inhaled will be reduced, carbon dioxide increases in the lungs. Plugging of the nose has also been practised by some students of Buteyko. A small piece of tissue is inserted into each nostril. This serves to reduce the amount of air passing through and therefore will increase carbon dioxide.

I have spoken with a number of people who claimed that they developed asthma solely from the breathing exercises that they were taught during yoga in Ireland. Unfortunately many of the exercises have become distorted along the way – possibly in an effort to facilitate Western lifestyles. The true intention of the exercises can in these circumstances be lost, and practices that may be harmful can be introduced. I suspect that this is what has happened in these cases.

Yoga is a complex subject. Many people practise it and feel that they get considerable health and peace of mind benefits as a result. I can only look at it from the point of view of whether or not it is likely to be of benefit to someone with an asthma problem who is trying to address an incorrect breathing pattern.

If it helps people to relax, and it also helps them to reduce their breathing, then there may well be a role for it.[6] The measure of success will be if it helps them to get their asthma under control.

Conclusion

Breathing exercises aimed at reversing hyperventilation have worked for me where nothing else ever has. I believe in it, and I want to help others to achieve what I have managed to achieve – permanent control of my asthma with no reliance on medication.

breathe right during physical activity

'A man's health can be judged by which he takes two at a time – pills or stairs.'

– Joan Welsh

The importance of exercise

It is important to note that depending on the severity of your condition, and on your general medical history, you may need to check with your doctor before starting a new exercise regime.

Physical exercise is essential for every asthma sufferer. In fact physical exercise and plenty of it is beneficial for everyone – asthma sufferer or not – but unfortunately the modern lifestyle very often encourages long periods of inactivity. Exercise should not be limited to young people or people involved in sport; it is beneficial to everyone provided that they exercise within their own limits. I have taught children as young as four and adults up to eighty-eight years old. The advice is the same to each and every one of them – spend as much time outdoors as possible and take some form of exercise.

People attending work-related training courses will be familiar with the mantra that applies to any newly learned skill: use it or lose it. This is as true for our bodies as for our minds and it is especially true for asthma sufferers.

The human body was designed to lead a physically active life, therefore continued good health and well-being requires some degree of exercise. Over the years research has consistently shown that, compared to those who take little or no exercise, people who exercise regularly are healthier, live longer, have greater inner calmness, are more content and cope better with life's stresses and strains.

Unfortunately, as asthma often limits physical capabilities, the tendency is to try to avoid asthma attacks by avoiding exercise. This has been proven in a number of studies that have shown people with asthma have lower cardiovascular fitness than those who do not have asthma.[1,2]

A major step towards improving asthma is to take plenty of exercise and to take it regularly, but to stay within individual physical capabilities when doing so. Many researchers have recommended this lifestyle practice for all children and adults with asthma.[3,4]

There are two big differences between our lifestyle and that of a couple of generations ago: they tended to eat less and more healthily and had a far more physically active lifestyle (even if they had never heard the phrase).

Nowadays we have fallen into a sedentary routine – one that is having a disastrous effect on the health of the nation. Few of us walk or cycle to work, we drive or are driven and few of us have jobs that require much serious physical effort. Many of us do take exercise during our free time but many more are addicted to TV and/or the pub culture.

Young people follow a similar pattern and in the educational rat race that is a by-product of the Irish points system there is less and less time given to sport or indeed any form of physical activity. However, educational research shows that a good balance between sporting activity and study is extremely beneficial for students.

Most of our day is spent sitting and, as if this wasn't enough for the body to contend with, we then add stress, smoking, overeating and eating inappropriately. It is no wonder that the population of the western world is becoming less and less healthy and, as a result, putting more and more pressure on national health services. As one commentator suggested: 'If it weren't for the fact that the TV set and the refrigerator are so far apart, some of us wouldn't get any exercise at all.'

Taking exercise that is appropriate for the body helps to strengthen the immune system, gives the body more energy and builds up strength. We need to exercise and those who suffer from asthma need it most.

What sort of exercise?

It seems that the answer to the question is: whatever sort of exercise you like. Commencing exercise after a long period of minimal physical activity requires a number of points to be considered first.

Go for something you like doing, or could get to like. If you're into record keeping, then by all means chart your progress, but it isn't essential. Just try to achieve a little more each week; you'll know yourself how you're doing.

Slow and steady is the way to go. Don't be too ambitious when starting off, but do try to progress week to week – walk, or cycle, jog or swim further, faster and for longer.

Exercise within your capabilities. Try not to miss a day – make your daily exercise routine a priority. Beware of over training, you won't enjoy it and it won't help you in the longer term. Get out into the open air whenever you can, it's healthier and also enjoying yourself will help you to feel better.

We should exercise because we enjoy it and because we feel better for it. Adopting the attitude that 'taking exercise is a drag' will make success difficult. Even if the physical activity is not enjoyable at first because it may represent a major lifestyle change, try to stick with it or perhaps try a different activity. Eventually it will become enjoyable; after all, it is what the body was designed for.

There are gyms all over the country and these are ideal during the winter, or when the weather is bad. However exercising outdoors beats any gym and there is a whole range of options in this field.

Life's greatest pleasures are often the simple ones. Walking in the peace of the Irish countryside, listening to the music that nature provides, is one. Introducing children to the everyday wonders of nature is the greatest gift they can be given. Help them to appreciate bird song or to watch out for native animals – rabbits, foxes, hares – going about their daily business. There are still busy ducks and majestic swans on the country's lakes and rivers and it is possible to still catch the occasional glimpse or hear the splash of a fish jumping. There are still bats here and there, not the vampire bats of the horror industry, but bats such as the Pipistrelle whose mission in life is the consumption of large quantities of midges. There is great and simple pleasure in the natural world for any age.

Depending on which part of the country you live in, it is possible to walk by the sea, along a river or canal bank, or by the shores of a lake and there are still country lanes not infested with speeding traffic. Alternatively just walk around your own town or city – you should be able to find somewhere to go and you may even have a park nearby.

If personal preference or necessity, or a sociable nature, means opting for the indoors alternative then a gym is the next best thing. The exercise bike is a good alternative to cycling on roads (and a lot safer), rowing machines are pleasant to use, climbing machines are easier on the joints than the treadmills, but there's a whole range of exercise options available.

Swimming proves very beneficial for people with asthma, and swimming is a topic that will be discussed later in the book.

Exercise is a very good and, in fact, essential element in controlling asthma. While exercise is very beneficial in temporarily increasing carbon dioxide levels and conditioning the body to accept a higher level, it does not change the underlying breathing pattern. Reduced breathing by relaxation is the only breathing exercise that will do this. For example, exercising diligently for an hour each day then spending the rest of the day going about with the mouth open causes the benefits accrued from the increased carbon dioxide to be lost.

Reducing the possibility of an attack during exercise

Estimates at the incidence of exercised induced bronchospasm are anything between eighty per cent and ninety per cent.[5]

Exercise-induced asthma (also known as EIA) occurs due to an increased volume of breathing brought about by the demands of physical effort. The theory generally accepted among researchers is that increased ventilation cools and dehydrates the airways. With increased ventilation, airways are required to condition a greater volume of air and this causes the dehydration and cooling effect. According to Anderson, the greater the volume of ventilation, the greater the loss of water and cooling of the airways and so the greater the severity of bronchoconstriction.[6]

Buteyko cites the loss of carbon dioxide as playing the primary role. If the volume of air being breathed is greater than is required by the metabolism, the airways narrow and asthma symptoms occur. When this happens, the amount of carbon dioxide being breathed out is greater than the amount the metabolism is producing. This results in activation of the body's defence mechanism as it constricts the airways to prevent the loss of carbon dioxide.

Buteyko's theory carries a lot of weight because during physical activity ventilation increases far more than it would at rest. However, when the control pause is sufficiently high, there are no symptoms during exercise due to the muscles producing plenty of carbon dioxide to counterbalance the increase of breathing. If EIA were caused solely by airway dehydration, then surely symptoms would occur regardless of the CP or degree of exercise? Another question worth asking is: if airway cooling, or drying, is the cause of EIA, then at what temperature or air moisture content could exercise be taken in order to prevent an attack? Would an attack occur if exercise were taken in a steam room, for example?

Quite possibly all theories have a validating argument but it does not matter which theory is correct. The most important thing to recognise is that overbreathing causes bronchoconstriction.

How do you know if you are exercising correctly?

You are exercising correctly if you can achieve the following: nasal breathing, an improved control pause and if you no longer require reliever medication prior to exercise.

Nasal breathing: It is of the utmost importance that all breathing is done only through the nose, and especially when the CP is low. This comes as quite a shock to most people because mouth breathing is so predominant in every activity, including walking. When the change to nasal breathing is first made, fitness levels will tend to dip below the normal level. However with continued nasal breathing this will soon correct itself. Research conducted with top athletes has shown that fitness levels will improve substantially within eight weeks if nasal breathing is maintained. It is essential in reducing exercise-induced asthma and it is advisable for people involved in sports to train at a more relaxed pace until they become accustomed to nasal breathing. Once the new regime becomes like second nature more intensive training can be undertaken.

Regardless of what type of exercise is being undertaken, if the need to breathe in through the mouth arises then the training is too intense. For chronically ill people, this can occur after just a few steps. For people who are physically fit this may not occur until after a few miles of jogging. As soon as the need to breathe in through the mouth arises, it is important to stop and relax, wait for a few minutes to catch a breath and only then proceed with the exercise once again. For this reason, walking in a park where there are plenty of seats is a good idea. This affords the opportunity to sit down on a bench and relax for a few moments whenever the need to breathe through the mouth occurs. In a matter of just a few weeks it should be possible to walk the entire distance without having to sit down and the route should be a lot easier to complete than previously.

It is often pointed out that nasal breathing can become quite pronounced and audible during even mild exercise. The body's requirement for air increases substantially with any exercise. As a result the breathing becomes louder and many people are conscious that other people can hear them breathing while they are out walking. This is only a temporary state and breathing will reduce as the levels of carbon dioxide increase. Whatever happens it is important not to revert to mouth breathing.

Reliever medication: Only take short-acting reliever medication if it is really needed; this is accepted medical practice. Never take reliever medication if it is not needed because it is easy to develop a subconscious dependence on quick-acting reliever medication. Quite often an inhaler is taken out of habit rather than need. At the same time, continue to have the reliever close to hand just in case it is required midway through training. It is proven that a tolerance to reliever medication occurs over a period of time and this can result in more and more puffs being needed to reduce symptoms.

Asthma is a defence mechanism to prevent the further loss of carbon dioxide. When the airways constrict this is the body's way of reducing hyperventilation. If five puffs of reliever medication are typically required during a football match, then the asthma is totally out of control. It would be far safer to reduce the intensity and/or duration of exercise until such a large dose of medication is no longer required.

Controlled breathing during sports: All this might seem to indicate that people with asthma won't be able to compete at the top level in their chosen sport but, in fact, nothing could be further from the truth. Everything that an individual can do with the aid of relievers can be done without the need for medication – as long as attention is paid to breathing.

It is relatively easy to combine controlled breathing with sport, with the exception of sports that require intensive bursts such as sprinting. For example, playing football should not present a problem if a gentle and gradual warm-up is performed first. Other steps to aid breathing can also be taken during the match. When the ball is elsewhere, breathe a little less than is required and when running for the ball try to keep breathing through the nose. If it gets to the stage where the need arises to breathe through the mouth, calm the breathing and switch to nasal breathing as soon as the ball has been passed. If the need to breathe through the mouth for long periods occurs, then it is better to stop playing football until such breathing becomes easier and it is possible to play at the desired level. Continuing to play while not breathing properly will not help people with asthma. So while playing try to ensure the breathing is not too deep and remember to observe the breathing pattern as much as possible.

Walking for half an hour every day is probably the best exercise for anyone who has not been taking regular exercise. Initially it may be best to walk alone rather than having to keep pace with someone else. Walking alone also avoids talking which promotes mouth breathing and increases hyperventilation. While walking, breathing should be reduced and again if at any time the need to deep breathe is experienced while walking or doing any exercise, then slow down and relax. Resist the urge to breathe through the mouth and, instead, stop and calm the breathing and when ready start walking again.

Those people whose asthma is severe and who can only walk around twenty paces should start by just walking fifteen paces and stopping. Breathing should be reduced and it is important never to push the body beyond the point where breathing cannot be controlled; to do so would be counter-productive and potentially dangerous. Don't be too con-cerned by needing to start at a very modest level; perseverance will result in being able to gradually walk further and further.

Coaches and trainers

It is a common misconception that big breathing is good for our health and this arises nowhere more than in the area of sport and training. Many coaches mistakenly believe that taking big breaths in through the nose and out through the mouth is beneficial and the theory is that toxins in the lungs will be removed by exhalation. Sports people can be seen in gyms around the country taking intentional big breaths as they lift weights and force a breath out through the mouth as the weight is relaxed. Instructors regularly advise during a warm down to breathe in through the nose and out through the mouth. Why is this bad habit so deeply ingrained despite the fact no one has ever benefited from it?

Big breathing in this manner not only reduces oxygenation of tissues due to the role of carbon dioxide as a catalyst for the release of oxygen, but may also contribute to dehydration. The nose contains turbinates and a mucus blanket that serves to remove moisture as air is exhaled from the body. To illustrate this, breathe out through your mouth onto a glass surface and check to see how much moisture content is left on the glass. Do this a second time, but this time breathe out through your nose. The amount of moisture left after the mouth breath is far greater than that left after the nose breath. A loss of moisture from the body contributes to dehydration, and dehydrated airways can be very sensitive to various stimuli.

Sports instructors who take the initiative and apply this therapy will notice a dramatic improvement in the fitness levels of all students, both those who suffer from asthma and those who don't. Reduced breathing has been taught to a number of people involved in various sports at the top level. In every situation, recovery times have improved, lactic acid build up has reduced, the pulse rate has been reduced and overall fitness levels have been improved. In an area of such competitive pressure where fractions of seconds can make the difference between winning and losing, athletes who apply this therapy will have an advantage over their peers.

Case Study One

Patrick McKeown, author of this book

During my college years, I never exercised or played any sports. In part this arose from a fear of asthma attacks, in part from laziness and in part because I had other fish to fry. When I tried to commence breath retraining I was a disaster. I could only do short walks; initially my maximum while maintaining nasal breathing was about half a mile which, for a young man, was disgraceful. I had to walk at a slow pace and whenever I was unable to maintain nasal breathing, I slowed down and rested until I could breathe comfortably again.

However, I persisted and each morning I got up half an hour early to take a walk down a country road near where I was living. I particularly enjoyed the freshness of the morning, the birds singing and being close to nature. My walk was an excellent start to the day, which before this would involve rushing straight from bed to the breakfast table and to my place of work. Furthermore, it was beneficial in reducing my symptoms for the remainder of the day.

After a few months, as my fitness levels improved and my need for reliever medication had decreased, I progressed on to the next stage of increasing my fitness levels, which was to enrol at a gym.

My first fitness assessment at the gym was rather poor, as my only form of exercise up to that point had been walking. However, my blood pressure and pulse rate were excellent despite my relatively poor fitness. I attended the gym three times every week for about half an hour each time. At first, I would spend ten minutes cycling on an exercise bike in a relaxed manner with controlled nasal breathing. After my cycle, I would spend about twenty minutes lifting small weights. My warm down would be a short cycle of about five minutes.

Gradually over the following months I progressed from cycling to gentle jogging on a treadmill. For the first ten minutes I would warm up by walking at an easy pace no greater than five kilometres per hour. For the next twenty minutes, I would jog with continued nasal breathing at about nine kilometres per hour. This would then be followed by a warm down lasting about five minutes.

It was a step-by-step process but I was enjoying it, because I knew I was doing something very worthwhile and positive. I also knew that I was making very steady progress and that provided me with great motivation.

These days I jog about four miles three nights a week – with nasal breathing. Nasal breathing during running can create a substantial air shortage and this can cause the mouth to open. If you find your mouth opening, raise your tongue to the roof of your mouth to help prevent the air escaping. This will often be an instinctive response to help maintain nasal breathing. While I'm exercising, I make sure that I don't push myself too hard, which would cause discomfort and that I feel well throughout. After exercise, I have more energy, a reduced appetite and a feeling of well-being. I also have a better control pause which should be the norm for anyone after a good exercise session.

To this day I have maintained my love of exercise and expect to have it for the rest of my life. I have never felt better and will never revert to my previously poor lifestyle. Most people who apply themselves diligently to regular exercise will continue because they know how good life is with it. They have good energy levels, good health and they also feel calm and good about themselves. Other people know that they should be exercising but due to laziness, do not devote any time to it. They then wonder why they are fatigued, why they are putting on weight that is difficult to shift and why they are sick. It will continue to be a downward spiral unless they take the time out to reflect on the current state of affairs.

This is an interesting little reminder from Edward Stanley: *'Those who think they have not time for bodily exercise will sooner or later have to find time for illness.'*

Case Study Two

Shane

There is no better example of the advantages of breathing therapy in sports than Shane. Despite having asthma Shane holds a Fourth Dan Black Belt in Tae Kwon Do and won the world championship in Open Martial Arts at his weight in 2002.

Shane's asthma, as is the case with very physically fit people, was only of a mild severity. His symptoms would be chest tightness experienced during training and matches. His medication intake was two or three puffs of Ventolin daily and this would increase during a competition. Although this amount of medication is quite small, it was something that Shane had needed for many years. In addition, like all sports people he was concerned with whether his asthma would get worse. He lived in the hope that his symptoms would reduce during the run up to a competitive match. In a way he was at the mercy of his asthma, and that was something he could have done without, especially during championship fights.

Shane attended a number of consultations and made good progress. He reduced his training for the first couple of weeks in order to become familiar with the concept of reduced breathing and applied the tape at night while focusing a lot of attention on his breathing during the day so that he would make the change quickly. Shane was a diligent and disciplined student who was always a pleasure to teach. After two weeks of practising reduced breathing, Shane received his due reward of having no need for reliever medication. It is now a year since Shane was taught this method and he has not used his medication since. His fitness level has now surpassed what it was before and the bonus is that he no longer requires any medication. He has also noticed an improvement in the fitness levels of his own students because he has incorporated many of the points into their regime.

What is the best exercise for people with asthma?

In every situation involving physical activity, if the breathing volume is too great the rate of carbon dioxide loss is more than what is being produced by metabolic activity. For people with asthma, this loss of carbon dioxide results in the body defending itself by constricting the airways. When choosing a sport, always consider the action of the defence mechanism as a result of overbreathing. Therefore, determining which sport is best is an individual choice based on both the current CP and ability.

No matter what sport or exercise is chosen, adhere to the following: be able to maintain control of your breathing at all times; be able to perform exercise with nasal breathing; feel good throughout the exercise, and enjoy it.

For example, the exercises quite often found to be most suitable are walking, jogging, cycling and lifting modest weights. Sports such as sprinting involve huge bursts of energy and require panting and mouth breathing. Cross country skiing has the highest incidence of asthma due to mouth breathing of very cold air which irritates hypersensitive airways.[7,8,9]

Swimming has always been regarded as an ideal sport for people with asthma with many sufferers competing at world-class levels.[10,11] This is believed by some to be the result of inhaling warm air during exercise.[12]

What many people don't realise is that swimming is practising reduced breathing exercises without realising it; it involves the movement of the arms and legs while at the same time breathing is restricted due to the head being under the water. This increases carbon dioxide levels because there is a combination of muscle activity and reduced breathing. Unfortunately, swimmers are not necessarily aware of the need to maintain correct breathing for the remainder of the day and so the benefits tend to be short lived. Of course, this will not prevent an attack occuring if a person is overbreathing during swimming.

Peter M. Donnelly, a respiratory professional, had a letter published in the *Lancet* entitled 'Exercise Induced asthma: The protective role of CO_2 during swimming'. In it he explained the role of swimming in producing a reduced minute volume of air and reduced symptoms in comparison with other sports. This occurred with all swimming styles except backstroke. Interestingly, a study during which athletes had complete protection from EIA during swimming showed that they did have a striking reduction in forced expiratory volume when they adopted running or cycling. This highlights the beneficial affects of swimming over other sports. He concludes that 'because end-tidal CO_2

tensions have not, as far as I am aware, been measured in asthmatics while swimming, the potentially important protective property of hypercapnia (high CO_2) may have been overlooked'.[10]

Summary of behaviour during sports and physical exercise

+ Exercise regularly and within your capabilities.
+ Walking or lifting light dumbbells/weights is excellent.
+ Nasal breathe during exercises. If you need to mouth breathe then you are pushing yourself too hard so stop for a rest and then begin again at a reduced pace.
+ Do not spend fourteen hours of your day sitting down like a lot of unhealthy people do.
+ Never mouth breathe.

chapter 6

food that helps, food that hurts

'Let your food be your medicine.'

– Hippocrates, 400 BC

Food plays a large part in our lives and so diet deserves special attention because it is certainly a contributory factor in causing overbreathing. The Asthma Care programme is seventy per cent retraining of breathing, fifteen per cent regular physical activity and fifteen per cent observation of diet. Buteyko's research indicates that food increases our breathing, some foods more than others, but water does not affect respiration.

Different food types

Our bodies can only absorb a small amount of energy in the form of vitamin D directly from the sun, but the remainder of our energy is absorbed from the food we eat. Food therefore will vary as a source of energy depending on how far it is removed from the sun. The only foods which receive this energy directly are fruit and vegetables. It is really no coincidence that this food group formed the staple part of people's diet for centuries. Meat is also a source of energy with animals absorbing the energy from the sun by eating the vegetation. We in turn eat the animals, thus indirectly receiving this energy.

Fruit and vegetables are of primary importance. A little meat is essential for good health, but for some people in the Western world it has become an obsession.

The third food group consists of processed food, including food which has been interfered with by man in the interests of productivity, efficiency and commercial gain. Processed food, the scourge of our planet, plays a big role in keeping hospital beds occupied by millions of patients each day.

Studies have consistently shown that those with asthma benefit from a diet rich in vegetables, fruit and whole grain and low in fat and alcohol consumption.[1] A healthy diet also helps improve breathing, achieving a higher control pause, and reducing asthma symptoms, leading to overall better health.

By carrying out breathing exercises properly you may experience a substantial reduction in appetite. This is because your body is better able to absorb nutrients from food due to increased oxygenation and improved blood supply to the gastrointestinal tract. Food then serves as a provider of essential nutrients as opposed to feeding disease. An old saying is: 'Of the food we eat, one third is for bodily requirements and two thirds is for the doctor'. Along with increased observation of breathing, pay attention to your body's requirement for food. When you do feel a reduction in appetite, do not force yourself to eat as this will slow down your progress. With breathing exercises and normalisation of CO_2, people who are overweight will reduce weight naturally, effortlessly and quickly.

Diet guidelines

✦ Do not overeat

Only eat when you feel hungry. Eating when you are not hungry means that your body uses energy in order to process food that it does not need. This leads to increased breathing and is not good for your health. Do not eat just because it is a particular time of the day. It is very important to adhere to this in order to help increase your control pause.

Stop eating when you feel you have had enough. Overeating will increase the risk factors for chronic degenerative disease such as cancer, diabetes, heart disease, and arthritic diseases. It has been well documented that reducing food intake will promote longevity of life. Reducing calorie intake while meeting your body's requirements of nutrients is the secret to a better and longer life. 'More die in the United States of too much food than too little'.[2]

Do not eat for a couple of hours before going to bed. If you have something to eat or a protein drink before you go to bed this will cause deep breathing during the night, will result in poor sleep and possible waking from symptoms. Sumo wrestlers intentionally have a large meal before they sleep in order to accumulate weight. The exact same process is happening to us, albeit unintentionally.

If your Control Pause is stubborn and you are experiencing difficulty increasing it even with regular physical activity then your food intake needs to be examined. For example semi-fasting or reducing meals by one per day can be very effective in increasing the Control Pause. During fasting or partial fasting dropping one meal per day will increase cortisol levels.

✦ Reduce your protein intake
Professor Buteyko found that high protein foods such as dairy, meat and eggs increase your volume of breathing. Independent of Buteyko, red meat is recognised as a contributory factor in inflammation. Research concludes that excessive protein is contributing to a higher prevalence of asthma in teenagers.[3] Have you ever noticed increased asthma symptoms or how tired you can be after eating a large dinner with meat? Professor Buteyko stated that although some people require protein, most people are better suited to a more vegetarian diet.

It should be a priority to reduce or eliminate dairy produce entirely from your diet because it can be mucus producing and may contribute to many allergies and breathing problems. Children with nasal congestion and runny noses often experience a great improvement when they stop drinking cow's milk. While this will not apply to all people in general, it does seem to apply to many people with asthma. Asian countries have very low dairy consumption due to lactose intolerance and their asthma rate is non existent compared with ours.[4]

If a person is lactose intolerant, dairy products are not a good source of calcium because the body is unable to absorb the calcium from milk sources.[5] If dairy is such a good provider, then why is osteoporosis often higher in countries with the highest dairy consumption?[6] Cow's milk is specially formulated and should be used only as nature intended which is to feed and develop calves. Milk is not the only food source to provide calcium. Good sources of calcium include kelp, turnip greens, rhubarb, broccoli, lambs kidney, tofu, tinned salmon with bones, baked beans, fortified oatmeal and other cereals, and all leafy green vegetables. Turnip greens provide an estimated twice as much calcium as milk.

A question often asked is this: what is there left to eat for breakfast if milk is eliminated from the diet? Your morning meal is to break your fast from the day before and to start your new day. Advertising and marketing gurus have unfortunately re-educated the masses to eat stale processed sugary foods for this important meal. Always remember that the foods which are widely advertised are usually processed foods. The best meal by far, which fed our ancestors for generations, is porridge. It provides essential fibre, energy and contains no additives, colouring or preservatives. Porridge cooked in the morning in water with a little honey is a good start to any day. If you are considering reducing your dairy intake, ensure that you eat green vegetables and consider calcium supplements, especially if you are taking steroids.

✦ Limit consumption of processed foods and stimulants

Consumption of processed foods should be limited. In the 1930s Dr Weston Price conducted an interesting study of traditional groups and their change to a more processed

westernised diet.[7] When the Gaelic people, living on the
Hebrides off the coast of Scotland, changed from their traditional diet of small sea foods and oatmeal to the modernised
diet of 'angel food cake, white bread and many white flour
commodities, marmalade, canned vegetables, sweetened
fruit juices, jams, and confections', first generation children
became mouth breathers and their immunity from diseases
of civilisation reduced dramatically. The traditional diets
were found to provide at least four times the minimum
requirement of nutrients, while modern diets did not meet
the minimum requirement.

Sugar affects your adrenals which produce your body's
natural source of steroid. Of sugary foods, chocolate has the
most harmful effect for any person with asthma. Sometimes
it may not be until the following day that symptoms are
experienced from the consumption of chocolate. Sugar raises
blood sugar levels and causes a depletion of essential minerals such as magnesium. Interestingly, 'desserts' spelled back-
wards is 'stressed'.

Little is known about the real nutritional content of
white bread. White flour contains little nutrition and
increases mucus production. To quote Dr Price's book *Nutrition and Physical Degeneration*: 'Modern white flour has had
approximately four fifths of the phosphorous and nearly all
of the vitamins removed by processing, in order to produce a
flour that can be shipped without becoming infested with
insect life. Tests showed that white bread was unable to
sustain insect life, while half a slice of whole rye bread was
totally consumed by bugs.' This begs the significant question:
how come white bread is not good enough for bugs to eat,

yet is good enough for humans to eat?

Black tea and especially **coffee** are regarded as stimulants. The group of asthma drugs known as Xantines are based on the same properties as coffee. These drugs are not now commonly used due to their many side effects. Coffee and tea will temporarily help you to breathe because they stimulate the adrenals and open up the airways in an extreme situation. The amounts needed to have any noticeable effect are large, but this will produce some unpleasant side effects and cause stress to the body in the long run. When Buteyko was asked if coffee was bad for you, his reply was: 'Try giving it to a cat'. He drew a lot of his conclusions from animals who instinctively know what, when and how much to eat. A person with sinus problems should avoid coffee altogether. Alternatives are herbal teas which are pleasant to drink and without any side effects. Some which are helpful for people with asthma in particular are ginger and lemon tea, and peppermint tea.

✦ Eat more fresh food

Fresh food is best. Canned food is not recommended due to the contamination of the food by aluminium packaging. Frozen vegetables, while not ideal, are a better source of prepared vegetables than canned. Best of all is **fresh fruit** and **vegetables** grown without the use of pesticides or chemical fertilisers. I remember, as a child, watching a woman in our local store who was searching for cabbages which had been attacked by slugs and other 'insects'. Her reasoning for this was that the cabbage which had been attacked by the insects had far less chemical on it. Chemicals increase your breathing rate because your body must eliminate this source of increased toxicity. Again, commercialisation and productivity take precedence over the health of the people.

It is beneficial to eat five portions of fresh vegetables and fruit per day, especially greens such as cabbage, broccoli, kale and kelp because these provide good sources of **magnesium** and **calcium**. Furthermore, vegetables do not promote the formation of mucus. Lightly cooking food and vegetables provides a richer source of nutrients and has less effect on breathing. However, the more raw the food, the less the effect it has on our breathing.

Ingredients such as **garlic, ginger, curry, onions** and **sea salt** are beneficial for asthma. Garlic, ginger and onions boost the immune system, thin mucus and are very helpful for people with respiratory complaints. Professor Buteyko also advocated using sea salt for cooking because it contains numerous essential minerals, thins mucus and is a natural anti-histamine. It is recommended that you drink a small amount of sea salt in warm water any time you have asthma symptoms and especially during the cleansing reaction.

Fruits which may **not be helpful** for people with asthma include oranges, grapefruits, lemons and limes as they are antigenic, i.e. they trigger an immune response. Drinking large amounts of orange juice each day may exacerbate symptoms. Bananas are mucus producing because they contain high potassium, and strawberries and raspberries increase histamine levels.

✦ Food intolerances

There are many foods to which you can be **intolerant** but usually eat every day. You may not notice the negative effect because there is a delayed reaction and symptoms run from one day into the next. Regular amounts of the offending food will ameliorate the effect of the initial consumption, resembling the alcoholic who consumes further quantities to obtain relief from his addiction.

The following foods commonly trigger symptoms: **milk, eggs, peanuts, soy, wheat, fish** and **shellfish.** Along with these are many **additives** such as **sulphites, Tartrazine,** and **monosodium glutamate.**[8]

Some foods can give you direct feedback on whether they are helping you or hurting you. For example, if your nose is totally clogged after drinking a cup of coffee – then coffee does not suit you. (It is debatable whether it suits anyone.)

Testing for food intolerance does require some detective work. Some indicators of food intolerance are foods that your parents are allergic to, foods you crave and foods you eat between meals. Crisps and chocolate are the most common items to fall into this category.

A good method of determining which foods you may be intolerant to is by eliminating them for a period of weeks. It is worth noting that if you cannot do without a food for twenty-one days, then you are very likely to be addicted to that food. For example, if you feel that milk exacerbates your symptoms, then for two weeks do not drink milk or consume any product which contains milk. By then you should have noticed an improvement in your condition if milk does not agree with you. If you do decide to reintroduce an offending food into your diet, be very careful because the reaction may be far greater following a period of withdrawal. It is advisable to speak with a nutritional expert before embarking on an elimination diet.

Other tests include missing your evening meal. On waking consume a small quantity of the suspect food. If your pulse rises more than ten beats fifteen minutes after eating, then consider eliminating this food from your diet and observe if there is an improvement in your condition.

Food guidelines summary

✦ Eat only when you feel hungry.
✦ Eat until you feel satisfied. Do not continue to eat because there is food left on your plate.
✦ Eat fruit and vegetables each day.
✦ Eat spices, curries, ginger, garlic, onions and sea salt.

Foods to limit in quantity are:

✦ Dairy and products containing dairy ingredients.
✦ Milk, yoghurt, cheese, Ice cream, cream soups, chocolate. (Please note that chocolate is by far the worst food to eat.)
✦ High protein foods such as beef, pork, chicken and eggs.
✦ Stimulants such as coffee, strong teas, alcohol, cocoa, soft fizzy drinks and drinking chocolate.
✦ Antigens such as citrus fruits, raspberries, strawberries, wheat and nuts.

Mucus producing foods are:

+ Dairy produce.
+ Chocolate.
+ Animal protein.
+ Processed foods such as white flour.
+ Coffee and alcoholic beverages.

Diet supplementation

Vitamin and mineral supplementation is recommended for people with asthma because hyperventilation causes the body to excrete some minerals such as magnesium, calcium and potassium in order to maintain PH. It is therefore necessary to replenish these because the loss of these minerals leads to further hyperventilation. Asthma causes chronic stress on the body so correct nutrient intake is vital.

The quality of food can be suspect and while a correct diet is a priority, it is also beneficial to supplement it with key minerals and vitamins. It is a fact that the increasing use of pesticides, chemicals on vegetation and feeding of animals with antibiotic and hormone laden food poisons our bodies with increased toxicity.

Magnesium, the natural bronchodilator

Scientists in the early 1950s reported that magnesium was a natural bronchodilator that relaxes smooth muscle and opens constricted airways without any side effects. Nowadays some intravenous magnesium sulphate is used as a partial treatment for attacks at a number of clinics in the U.S.[9,10,11]

The typical Western world processed diet contains very low levels of magnesium. A deficiency of magnesium will further perpetuate hyperventilation. Another reason for magnesium deficiency is intense farming practices. Mineral levels have fallen over the past fifty years due to continued harvesting. Only nitrogen, phosphorous and potassium are replaced in order to produce higher yields. My experience of taking magnesium either in diet or supplement has been very helpful in reducing hyperventilation and increasing my control pause.

I spoke with a number of people who test mineral and vitamin levels among their patients and all concluded that magnesium was very low in most asthmatics. Magnesium also helps to stabilise the Mast cell producing anti-inflammatory effects.[12]

One Nottingham study has shown a relationship between increased peak flow readings and magnesium intake. This also correlated with decreased airway reactivity to methacholine challenge.[13] Another study points to a possible role for magnesium because of its bronchodilating effect in the treatment of asthma.[14]

Magnesium can be purchased in most health stores. The best form is liquid because it's absorbed better by the body, but magnesium tablets in chalk form are very beneficial. Personally, I use a magnesium, calcium and zinc combination.

Natural sources of magnesium include sea salt, kelp, sunflower seeds, spinach, avocado, barley, almonds, Brazil nuts, oysters, sunflower seeds, whole grains, beans and dark leafy vegetables. Supplement magnesium according to recommended daily amounts (RDA) as stated by manufacturers.

Vitamin B5, commonly known as Pantothenic acid

Pantothenic acid stimulates the adrenals and is involved in the production of cortisone. Allergies, adrenal exhaustion or upper respiratory infections are often a sign of B5 deficiency because the adrenals become weak and compromised. Other benefits from vitamin B5 include reducing the toxic effects from antibiotics. Good sources include corn, eggs, heart, kidney, legumes, lentils, liver, lobster, molasses, peanuts, peas, rice, soybeans, sunflower seeds, vegetables, wheat germ, and whole grain cereals.

Omega-3 fatty acids

Omega-3 fatty acids are a natural anti-inflammatory that quiet down key inflammatory cells such as neutrophils and prostaglandin. Essential fatty acids, when taken over time, work like cortisone without the side effects. There have been mixed results in studies of Omega-3 and this seems to be related to the length of the study, with longer trials producing more conclusive results.[15,16,17]

The time frame to take Omega-3 is for a minimum of ten weeks to reduce inflammation. Flaxseed oil, hemp oil or Evening Primrose oil are good forms of Omega-3 and are recommended more than fish oil due to the high mercury content of the seas. Massaging hemp oil into areas of the skin affected by eczema offers substantial relief.

One word of caution: people who are sensitive to aspirin may experience an increase of asthma symptoms. If you do notice a deterioration, stop taking Omega-3 immediately.

The list of vitamins and minerals above are those I find, from available research, to be the most effective. Magnesium is a natural bronchodilator, Panthothenic acid helps rebuild the adrenals and Omega-3 is a natural anti-inflammatory. There is an exhaustive list of vitamins and minerals recommended for asthma and it would not be beneficial or practical to take them all. If you only wish to take one of these then I recommend magnesium. I also suggest that you have echinacea on standby should the need ever arise. Multivitamins are very helpful but the levels are too low to be of any benefit. Speak to someone who is knowledgeable at your health store to seek further information regarding supplements for children and what products are available.

Water

Water makes up over seventy per cent of your body and it's the single most important constituent of your diet. You consume water directly by drinking it and indirectly from your diet. You lose water each day through perspiration, breathing, and elimination of waste. It is vital therefore to replenish this water loss because dehydration causes an increase of histamine levels, causing inflammation and swelling of the airway walls.

To help reduce water loss breathe only through your nose. On average we take eighteen thousand breaths over a twenty-four hour period, with this figure increasing substantially for a person with asthma. One of the functions of your nose is to trap moisture carried in the air on the out breath.

The second step is to reduce the group of drinks containing caffeine and alcohol. These drinks are diuretics and, while they contain water, they promote dehydration because the kidneys flush out additional water. More water leaves the body than is contained in the drink, yet many people believe that tea is a good source of water. Unfortunately it isn't and if you feel unable to reduce your tea consumption, then increase your pure water intake to counteract this loss.

The third step is to eat a diet high in water content. People who live on a water-rich diet of fruit and vegetables are free from obesity and illness and often live well in excess of one hundred years. A water-rich diet is the secret to better health and longevity.

The amount of water you need depends on the type of lifestyle you lead. A person who is involved in physical activity will have a greater requirement. Likewise, it is dependent on the type of diet. If you eat a water-rich diet then the requirement to drink water is reduced.

In the medical world, there are mixed beliefs about whether thirst alone is a good indicator of the need for water. Nutritional experts suggest a daily water intake of six to eight glasses. Using this as a guide, and taking into account your individual lifestyle and diet, you can estimate individual requirements. If your lifestyle is to drink ten cups of tea a day and eat a processed food diet, then you are chronically dehydrated.

With asthma, the key point to remember is that the need for water is increased because dehydration leads to histamine production and thickened mucus. A quarter to a half-teaspoon of sea salt dissolved in warm water serves as a natural antihistamine, thins out mucus and can, in as little as fifteen minutes, reduce asthma symptoms.

To keep your body well hydrated, adults should drink about eight glasses of water per day and make a conscious effort to maintain consistent intake.

Everyone needs water to regulate body temperature, aid respiration, transport nutrients, aid elimination of waste, provide lubrication, and give tissues their structure.

what's your trigger?

'When your Control Pause is forty seconds, you will have no more questions concerning triggers.'

What is more important – correct breathing or elimination of triggers? This chapter is designed to provide some useful tips on reducing your exposure to certain triggers. The main cause of your asthma is overbreathing and triggers simply bring on symptoms when your immune system is hypersensitive to them.

When you breathe correctly you will have no adverse reaction to triggers. With this in mind your priority should be to change your breathing. Allocate ninety-five per cent of your attention to your breathing and only five per cent to eliminating the triggers. If you eliminate all your triggers but have done nothing to address your breathing, you will still have asthma. If you correct your breathing and do nothing about your triggers, your asthma will still improve immensely.

On the road to recovery

A trigger is anything which can cause symptoms to arise so if you have inherited bronchospasm and overbreathe, pollen, dust mites, pollution, smoke, stress and other factors can trigger your asthma attack.

The control pause, the main indicator of the state of your asthma, tells you whether it is improving or deteriorating. In treating asthma you should adopt a holistic approach, tailored to your individual needs and taking lifestyle factors into consideration. Very few physicians give advice on breathing through the nose, diet, exercise, or any other natural action which can be implemented for the treatment of asthma. Generally, you go to your doctor with the intention of receiving medication. I feel this is a failure of our medical system because both patients and doctors have too much of a reliance on medication, on the quick fix. This quick fix is life-long and it is usual to expect that the amount of medication increases rather than decreases over time. Some children do 'grow' out of asthma but all too often this comes back later in life.

Sometimes asthma triggers can be quite obvious. If you experience increased nasal congestion or wheezing after making beds, doing housework, hoovering, folding clothes or any other household chore, then it is very likely that you are allergic to dust mites. Knowing the trigger is the first step in dealing with it. Other very common triggers include pollen, moulds and animal dander.

What are the signs of an allergy?

+ Frequent sneezing, watery eyes and cold-like symptoms.
+ A crease above the tip of the nose caused by regular upward wiping of the nose (allergic salute).
+ Coughing, wheezing and other asthma symptoms.
+ Dark circles under your eyes as a result of increased blood flow to the sinuses.

What are the more common triggers?

+ Dust
+ Moulds
+ Pets
+ Pollen
+ Air pollutants
+ Tobacco smoke
+ Exercise
+ Weather
+ Stress

Dust

Household dust contains various particles including microscopic creatures known as dust mites. It is estimated that thirty thousand of these tiny creatures can live in one ounce of dust found in every fabric and furnishing. It is not the actual dust mites that are the problem but the droppings. Dust mites live primarily by consuming human skin scales which we shed in relatively large quantities each day. They do not feed off us directly but off the skin we shed. Not all asthma sufferers have an allergy to the dust mite so a little observation is necessary. For example, do you have increased symptoms after any of the following:

+ Making beds?
+ Vacuuming?
+ Spending time in houses with large areas of carpets?
+ Sleeping on old beds?
+ Folding clothes?
+ Exposure to dust from any source?

Dust mites thrive indoors in warm and damp houses. The greater the amount of newspapers, books, fabric furnishings, carpets and curtains, the greater the number of mites. However, no matter how clean and tidy a house is, it is never possible to eliminate dust mites completely. A hospital environment is probably the most suitable for avoiding dust mites but it's not practical to live in a hospital all the time. Living in a cocoon in order to avoid allergens is simply not feasible. Correct breathing and a little detective work will be of great assistance in reducing the possibility of dust mites being one of your triggers.

Beds are the greatest potential source of allergen due to a plentiful supply of skin scales and humidity from perspiration.

If you are allergic to dust, it is helpful to implement the following:

+ Purchase a new bed if the mattress is old.
+ Use anti-mite or allergen impermeable covers on mattresses/ pillows and put tape on seams to reduce dust mite escaping. It is estimated that sixty-six per cent of all

dust mites throughout the house reside in our beds. While lying down we shed skin scales and sweat. This creates an ideal environment to house a population of dust mites.[1]

+ Wash bedclothes regularly at a temperature of sixty degrees or higher. Temperatures must be greater than fifty-five degrees in order to kill dust mites.[2]

+ It is better if children do not sleep in the lower half of a bunk bed because constant movement of the top mattress will stir up mites.

+ Soft toys harbour a lot of dust mites. Freeze toys for one day each week prior to washing.

+ Remove pot plants and fish tanks because they are sources of humidity.

+ Do not dry clothes on radiators, especially in the bedroom.

+ When dusting use a damp cloth to prevent dust from rising.

+ If you are allergic to dust, do not work in a dusty environment. Always wear a dust mask or ask someone else to carry out chores that may expose you to dust.

+ Use a Dyson vacuum cleaner or one that retains air.

+ Have wooden floors rather than carpets in bedrooms. Carpet can trap large amounts of dust mites, skin, mould spores, pet dander and any chemicals which have been used in carpet cleaning.

+ Direct sun-light is one of the most effective ways of reducing dust mites on rugs. Placing rugs upside down for a number of hours under direct sunlight will kill all dust mites and mite eggs.

+ Replace heavy curtains with light material.
+ If the bedroom is excessively damp, consider using a dehumidifier which will reduce the moisture content of the air. If the air is excessively dry, it can irritate sinuses and the respiratory system.

Household dust contains a varied assortment of potentially allergenic particles including:

+ Pollens
+ Moulds
+ Animal dander
+ Insect parts
+ Flakes of human skin

Moulds

Moulds are found indoors and outdoors depending on environmental conditions. Moulds, tiny unseen microscopic spores which float in the air, are produced by different forms of fungi which can be recognised by their dark colour and often furry-like appearance. They thrive in damp and wet conditions. We breathe in millions of mould spores when we are in a mouldy environment and this will trigger an asthma attack for some people.

Do you experience symptoms during any of the following situations:

+ Damp rainy days.
+ Autumn/Winter months.
+ Exposure to rotten vegetation, leaves, grass, hay or food.
+ Handling damp mildewed clothes.
+ Spending time in old houses with rising damp.
+ Spending time in bathrooms with black mould on shower curtains and/or ceiling.

Moulds need a damp environment to appear and survive so it's helpful to adopt measures to maintain as dry a home as possible. These measures will help:

+ Ventilate your house thoroughly, especially on dry days.
+ Remove pot plants and fish tanks because they are sources of humidity.
+ Do not dry clothes on radiators, especially in the bedroom.
+ Ventilate bathrooms, especially en-suites.
+ Use undiluted bleach to clean any mouldy surfaces. Check window frames, shower curtains, bathroom ceilings, kitchen walls, kitchen counter tops, bedrooms with en-suite bathrooms, and old furniture.
+ If rooms in your house are excessively damp, then you may need to consider having the walls dry lined. As a temporary measure, a dehumidifier can be used to reduce the moisture content of the air.
+ Areas along the side of your house which receive very little direct sunlight may have an abundance of moulds. There are various outdoor anti-fungal products available to control this.

Pets

People believe that animal allergies are caused by fur or feathers, but in fact allergies arise from proteins left from saliva after the animal licks its fur during the cleaning routine. When the saliva dries, it breaks up into tiny particles which become airborne. Animal dander consists of very tiny particles naked to the human eye and can linger on for weeks and months after the pet is gone.

Pets producing the most allergen are cats and regular washing does little to help the situation as a new supply is produced very quickly.

I receive regular queries from people asking if pets are a trigger. A little observation on your part will help answer this question.

For example, do you experience symptoms after:

+ Handling or petting an animal?
+ Visiting a house where an animal is kept indoors?
+ Visiting pet stores?

Does your asthma improve if you have not been near your pets for a period of time?

The best advice is to keep animals outdoors. If it is essential for the pet to remain indoors, ventilate the house thoroughly and keep the pet out of the bedroom. Wash your hands after you handle an animal to avoid transfer of dander from your hand to your mouth and nose.

Pollen

In Spring, Summer and Autumn, tiny particles are released into the wind from flowers, grass, trees and plants and are carried on air currents for the purpose of fertilisation. Many of these particles do not reach their intended destination and instead enter human airways, often acting as a trigger for asthma.

Pollen, because it is so widespread, is almost impossible to avoid and even staying indoors may not help because it is carried through vents, on clothes and enters buildings whenever doors are opened. Pollen can be found very far out to sea and at vast heights, giving an indication of the distance it can travel.

Some countries with hot climates can have a high pollen count for the entire twelve months of the year, other countries for a particular season. In Britain and Ireland, Spring and Summer are usually the worst time for high pollen counts. The main instigators of airborne pollen are grasses, trees and weeds which produce light microscopic particles easily carried by air currents. It is not the pollen from brightly coloured flowers that is a trigger, because insects and not the wind carry the pollen from plant to plant.

A pollen count is a measure of the amount of pollen in the air in a particular area at a certain time. Pollen counts tend to be highest on warm, dry, breezy days and lowest during cold, wet days.

Do you experience symptoms on:

+ Hot, dry Summer days?

✦ Being near hay, mowed lawns, golf courses or football pitches?

✦ Days with a high pollen count (pollen counts are often highest in the morning)?

✦ Being outdoors during some seasons?

Measures to reduce pollen exposure:

✦ Keep all doors and windows closed.

✦ Wear sunglasses.

✦ Dry clothes with a dryer. Do not leave them outdoors where they can trap a large amount of pollen.

✦ Stay away from newly mowed lawns, farms or other sources of pollen.

Air pollutants and tobacco smoke

Many studies have been undertaken which point to a link between asthma and air pollutants. However, while air pollutants can be a trigger, they are certainly not the cause. New Zealand, Australia and Ireland, where the pollution levels are not high, have the highest incidences of asthma in the world. Other countries in South East Asia and Eastern Europe are very heavily polluted yet the rate of asthma is relatively low.

An interesting study was carried out in the former East Germany prior to unification with West Germany. Pollution levels were significantly higher in the Eastern part yet asthma was significantly lower. It was only when East Germany started adopting the practices of a Western lifestyle that asthma started to increase.[3] Eating processed foods, increased temperatures of houses, over-eating, lack of physical exercise and stress, for example, cause overbreathing and overbreathing is causing asthma.

Pollution, including cigarette smoke, contains noxious particles and exposure to it is not good for any person. People with asthma find it difficult to visit countries such as Spain where smoking is very common. They are also unable to enter smoky buildings such as pubs or restaurants due to the likelihood of having an attack.

According to some estimates about ten per cent of people with asthma continue to smoke. Not only does a person who smokes take big breaths, they also intentionally bring highly poisonous pollutants into their airways. Smoking immobilises cilia, the tiny hair like structures that form our defence against foreign particles entering the airways.[4] These foreign particles are trapped by the thin layer of mucus which rests on the cilia. This mucus is then brushed in an upward motion to the throat where it is swallowed. It is thought that one cigarette immobilises cilia for one hour. Therefore a person who smokes twenty cigarettes a day will have constant immobilisation of cilia, thereby reducing their defensive capabilities.

Everyone, especially people with asthma, should be encouraged to give up cigarettes. While you are giving up smoking, practise reduced breathing and maintain low stress levels. Stress may increase a little during the rehabilitation phase and an increase in stress leads to an increase in breathing which leads to an increase in asthma. Reduced breathing will allow you to remain calmer because the excitability of your brain cells will be reduced. When under stress, bring attention inside your body and reduce your breathing. Giving up cigarettes requires a combination of approaches. Try reading Allen Carr's book entitled *The Only Way to Stop Smoking*, watch his video and at the same time attend a hypnotist to have the addiction removed from your subconscious. I am not in favour of patches, chewing gum or switching to cigars because they involve replacing one form of nicotine with another. In my experience people become just as addicted to patches or nicotine chewing gum as they did cigarettes. Eventually, most people sense they are addicted to the replacement and therefore will just revert to the original bad habit.

Exercise

For the majority of people, exercise can induce asthma giving spasm like symptoms, wheezing, breathlessness and coughing. However, physical exercise is important to help produce carbon dioxide and so people with asthma should do some form of exercise. Due to a fear of having an attack most people avoid it. This leads to a vicious circle of poor fitness levels and more asthma symptoms.

For more detailed information on correct breathing during exercise, refer again to chapter five.

Weather

Weather is certainly a trigger but the cause is hyperventilation. If a person with bronchospasm hyperventilates in Africa, then they will have asthma. It doesn't matter where you live, the question is this: are you big breathing? Australia has a beautiful climate, yet the incidence of asthma is high, indicating that warm weather does not have a profound effect.

Weather types and changes are a frequent trigger of asthma. People whose asthma is triggered by weather generally experience greater symptoms on wet, damp days. Ireland is especially prone to wet weather and so a lot of asthmatics are affected.

It is quite possible that damp and foggy weather involving a drop of atmospheric pressure results in a greater loss of carbon dioxide from the body due to the pressure difference. It is very common for people to wake up on a wet day feeling miserable, drained of energy with increased symptoms and a blocked stuffy nose.

Other explanations of how damp days increase symptoms may be the tendency to remain indoors and therefore be exposed to greater concentrations of dust mites which can be a trigger for many people. Wet days also result in a greater amount of moulds.

When I started practising breath retraining I experienced a period of weeks during which I felt good and then I woke up feeling terrible on other days. There was a direct relationship between the weather and my symptoms. I also knew that when I lived in Sweden and Australia, my symptoms decreased somewhat.

Weather continued to be a trigger for me for a number of months and sometimes I resigned myself to the fact that my symptoms would be worse on a damp day. Over time however, as my control pause continued to increase, damp weather as a trigger decreased. Now damp weather has very little effect on me.

Another trigger is a drop in temperature. For some people this may be as slight as a decrease of a couple of degrees. Changes in temperatures can act as a shock to the body and can contribute to hyperventilation. One way to reduce this is to consciously control breathing as you enter a decreased temperature. For example, if you are entering a cold room, practise reduced breathing. Make sure that you do not overbreathe.

You may have noticed that when people jump into a swimming pool, river or sea, they will start to hyperventilate if the water is cold. The cold water is a stress which increases breathing. If you are about to swim or take a cold shower, immerse yourself very gradually. Start by immersing your feet for about ten seconds, then let the water up to your knees for another ten seconds, then your waistline. At this point it is helpful to splash water onto your chest a number of times before immersing fully. Healthy people will be far better able to tolerate colder water than unhealthy people. A cold shower is very beneficial but only when you are already healthy.

Cold air is known to be a trigger. For example, the sport with the greatest incidence of asthma is cross-country skiing. This may be caused by mouth-breathing excessively dry cold air. The airways are a warm moist environment and therefore it is important that the air inhaled meets this condition. New research, as discussed by Professor Jonathan Brostoff in his book, *Asthma, The Complete Guide*, indicates that it may not be inhaling cold air which causes symptoms but instead the effect of cold air on the face. This would indicate that a shock is produced from the face being exposed to cold air. To avoid this shock, wear a hat or scarf and keep your face warm. Continuous breathing through the nose will also condition the air better and maintain more correct carbon dioxide levels. More than likely, triggers from cold air are caused by both thermal shock and hypersensitive airways which are further irritated by cold dry air.

Windy days are another factor. Trying to breathe on a windy day is like trying to breathe with a pillow pressed over your face and this can be experienced by both asthmatics and non-asthmatics alike. For people with asthma, this may increase their apprehension and therefore create a slight panic effect. Of course, this would increase breathing, resulting in increased symptoms.

Generally, to minimise the effects from weather, wear a hat or scarf while in cold places and reduce your breathing to avoid hyperventilation induced by thermal shock of any kind.

Stress

Stress, a condition of the Western world, increases with the pace of life. According to the famous physiologist Walter Cannon, stress activates the fight or flight response. Meeting deadlines, financial pressures, pressure of rearing children, doing well in our work and many other factors add to stress levels.

Long term stress is exhausting and it is known to result in many illnesses including asthma. It increases breathing, causing a loss of carbon dioxide, and resets the respiratory centre in the brain to a lower level. Many people with asthma are aware that their symptoms increase when their stress levels rise. Many more people, especially those with late onset asthma, developed it as a result of stress.

Stress in children?

Many theories exist on this subject. One is that asthma often develops as a result of the child being away from their mother for a period of time. It is interesting that emotions, anxiety or a feeling of being upset do increase breathing. Over time, this increase of breathing can be sustained, leading to the development or exacerbation of asthma.

Another observation is that some children may wittingly throw a tantrum which will increase their breathing and start an attack. They know that their attack will bring them attention. This does not apply to all children but I have experienced it on a number of occasions. In this situation, an attack is still serious regardless of how it happened. If you feel that your child may bring on the attack to attract your attention, then explain your observation and teach them to reduce their breathing when they are upset. When they are upset, remind them to keep their mouth closed and about the effect that their emotions are having on their breathing. Children have little stresses of their own and these in turn can influence their asthma.

Does stress affect children? My view is that of course it does. While the stresses may be in a different context to ours, they do exist. Children learn to adapt in an environment with many other children. A quiet child can be subject to the bullying antics of another child. A teacher may be hard on pupils, resulting in stress. The child has the pressure to keep up at school and cope with being on time, for example. Yes, children do have little stresses and recognising this is a help, especially if the stress is influencing their breathing. Teach them to control their breathing any time they are under stress and always encourage them to partake in physical activity.

Managing stress

There are a number of techniques available to help with managing stress. It is most important to control your breathing during stress. Watch other people who are stressed and listen to their breathing. Notice that they will be mouth-breathing with a very large volume and this increase in breathing will further increase stress levels.

Paying attention to your breathing is a very calming and meditative practice. It's time you devote to yourself by focusing attention inside to feel the life within. It's very helpful to take your attention off your thoughts on a regular basis. Feel the underlying field of stillness, let everything slow down for a few moments and follow your breath. See your breath, feel your breath and practice reduced breathing by relaxation. A calm mind will always be more productive than an erratic or worried one. If you do find yourself getting stressed, bring your attention back to your breathing as quickly as you can and enter the realm of peace. Thoughts may still arise but don't fight them in any way. Instead, recognise them and bring your attention back to your breathing.

This is a very helpful exercise and one which I use on a daily basis. Have you ever noticed how much easier it is to deal with anything when the mind is calm? The benefits of reducing thought and bringing attention to your breathing is that it allows true intelligence and ideas to rise to the surface.

It has been estimated that we generate fifty-three thousand thoughts per day and psychologists estimate that ninety-eight per cent of these are repetitive and useless. Most creative and unique ideas stem from a period of no thought. Most stress arises from thought.

Reduce the amount of trigger you are inhaling

Correct breathing improves your immune system, resulting in a significant reduction in the effect that a trigger will have. In addition, many millions of trigger particles are inhaled when you overbreathe.

When you are more aware of your breathing, nasal breathing predominates and the volume of air inhaled is reduced, resulting in a considerable reduction in the amount of trigger entering the airways. This alone will reduce the effect from exposure to triggers.

Always try to avoid the trigger. When exposed to dust, smoke, irritants, deodorants, pollution, do the following:

+ Breathe in.
+ Breathe out.
+ Hold your breath and walk away from the trigger.
+ Reduce your breathing.

The purpose of this is to raise your defence capabilities and also to inhale far fewer allergic particles.

Psychological element of asthma

During the 1960s, intrinsic asthma was the term used to describe asthma which had no known trigger. It was generally thought that because there was no known trigger, symptoms resulted from psychological factors, that it was all in the head. This attached a stigma to having asthma which only served to increase anxiety levels for many people.

Another factor involved, from a psychological point of view, is that of conditioning. Having repeated attacks from exposure to a trigger conditions the body to expect an attack each time the trigger is present. This response develops over time and the airways constrict, not just from the trigger itself, but from the psychological expectation of an attack. For example, a person who experiences an attack whenever they are exposed to cats can often have symptoms merely by just seeing a cat on the television.

This works in two ways. Firstly, stress levels rise on seeing the trigger and therefore breathing increases. Secondly, because the body is conditioned to have an attack from the presence of a trigger, airways will automatically constrict. For some people, merely imagining a trigger will start symptoms.

Psychologists claim it takes just twenty-one days for a conditioned response to be replaced with different behaviour. Now that you are aware of how your asthma is caused and how to reverse it, your anxiety levels will decrease and you will consciously replace the conditioned response with a different behaviour. Always remember that it is not the dust mites or smoke that is causing your asthma, instead it is your overbreathing, so work to reduce your overbreathing.

know your medication

'The best and most efficient pharmacy is within your own system.'
— Robert C. Peale

Given the number of people who have asthma, one could question whether Mother Nature has made a fundamental error in the airways of a large number of people. The truth is, it is quite likely she hasn't and that asthma is quite simply a defence or protection mechanism. Removing the stimulants that activate this defence mechanism is the first step on the road to taking control of the condition.

Although medication occupies a very important place in the treatment of asthma – everyone with the condition, regardless of age or severity of symptoms, should at least try natural measures to alleviate asthma. All drugs have side effects and every opportunity should be seized to minimise the dosage required. Natural measures such as contained in this book have been proven to reduce the amount of medication required and the very fact that you are reading this book indicates this is an approach you take seriously.

Medication for the treatment of asthma can be broadly divided into two groups namely reliever (bronchodilator) and preventer (steroid).

Reliever medication

Reliever medication is taken, as the name would imply, to obtain relief from symptoms. This is an important distinction from preventer medication taken to stop the symptoms from arising in the first place. The most popular form of reliever medication is the inhaler which will be familiar to most people; however it can also come in the form of a tablet or syrup. Reliever inhalers are easily recognisable by their blue, grey or green colour.

There are two types of reliever medication and they vary by how long the drug keeps the airways open. The most popular type of inhaler, which is known to everyone with asthma, is a short-acting reliever inhaler known as a beta2Agonist. This is taken only when needed and the effects last for three to four hours. Commonly prescribed short-acting relievers are Ventolin, Salamol and Bricanyl.

The drug and brand names of short-acting relievers are: Salbutamol commonly known as Ventolin, Salamol, Aerolin and Salbulin as well as Terbutaline that is commonly known as Bricanyl.

The second type of reliever inhaler is longer acting and keeps the airways open for about twelve hours. It is taken at regular times, usually in the morning and at night, and is marketed as Oxis, Serevent and Spireva.

The drug and brand names of long-acting relievers are: Salmeterol, commonly known as Serevent, and Eformoterol, commonly known as Oxis and Foradil.

Short acting reliever guidelines

This medication should be taken on a need-only basis to overcome attacks.[1] Try not to take reliever medication solely out of habit. Ensure that the inhaler is needed instead of instinctively reaching for it at the slightest hint of symptoms. If the symptoms are minor, try to stop the oncoming attack by using reduced breathing. If this does not stop the attack after five minutes, then take reliever medication. If the symptoms are severe, reliever medication should be taken immediately.

Try taking only one puff of the reliever inhaler each time. Professor Buteyko recommends taking one puff and waiting for the medication to take effect, which should happen within five minutes. If another puff is needed it should be taken at this stage. There is no point in taking two puffs of reliever medication when only one is needed. Steroids are different however and should be used according to the prescription and never altered without a doctor's consent.

Long-acting bronchodilators (relievers)

These inhalers keep the airways open for several hours and are taken once every twelve hours. They are prescribed for use on a regular basis, two puffs at a time, but should NEVER be used for emergencies. People have been known to die from taking long-acting relievers for symptomatic relief.

One of the shortfalls of reliever medication (bronchodilators) is that it does not cure asthma. No matter what dose is taken today it will make no difference to what symptoms are experienced tomorrow.

Reliever medication also causes hyperventilation. It forces the airways open and because the underlying hyperventilation is not addressed, the body will mount an even greater defence to prevent a further loss of carbon dioxide. Tolerance develops and the amount of reliever medication required to maintain control increases as the person gets older.

The side effects of bronchodilators can include: hyperventilation, hyperactivity, muscle tremors (often felt as a shaking of the hands), restlessness, dizziness, headaches, palpitations or gastrointestinal upsets.

Preventer medication

Preventer medication is predominantly steroid based and must be taken all the time, according to a doctor's instructions. Preventers come in red, brown or orange inhalers. Commonly used preventer medications are Flixotide, Becotide and Pulmicort.

Steroids (preventers) are the most effective anti-inflammatory drugs but they do not give immediate relief and their true worth only emerges with continuous use. A common mistake is to completely stop taking the preventer medication when fewer symptoms are experienced. In this case the asthma will slowly worsen over seven to twenty-one days, the need for a reliever will increase and this can result in a serious, uncontrolled asthma attack.

Steroids reduce inflammation which is the main compo-
nent of asthma[2] but they do not cure the underlying disease.

It is important to note that preventative medication
should never be stopped or reduced without consulting a
doctor first.

The drug and brand names of inhaled steroids are:
Beclomethasone Dipropionate 50, 100, 200, 250, 400 micrograms, commonly known as Becotide, Beclazone, Becloforte,
Aerobec, Filair and Qvar; Budesonide that is commonly
known as Pulmicort 100, 200, 400 micrograms and Fluticasone Propionate that is commonly known as Flixotide 25, 50,
125, 250.

Fluticasone is as effective as Beclomethasone Dipropionate and Budesonide at half the dose when given by equivalent delivery systems.[3,4,5]

Side effects at regular doses can include: candida (oral
thrush), inflammation of the tongue, a hoarse voice (dyspho-
nia) or easy bruising.

To reduce the side effects from a steroid inhaler the
mouth should be washed and rinsed after taking the inhaler
with the rinse water spat out to avoid swallowing any further
steroid. Using a large volume spacer will reduce the likelihood
of steroid being deposited in the mouth. This is also advised
for children as they may have a poor inhaler technique.

What is a low or high dosage?

The following table gives an indication of the relative dosage
of intake for Beclomethasone or Budesonide. As Fluticasone

Adults and children over five years old	Dosage of Beclomethasone or Budesonide
Low dose	100 to 400 mcg per day
Moderate dose	500-800 mcg per day
High dose	More than 800 mcg per day
Children under five years old	
Low dose	Less than 200 mcg per day
Moderate dose	250-400 mcg per day
High dose	More than 500 mcg per day

is double the strength of the amounts below, halve the figures to determine the relative dosage. For example, a moderate dose of Flixotide for adults is 250 to 400 mcg per day.

The drug and brand names of oral steroids include: Prednisolone 1, 5 and 25 mg tablets that are commonly known as Deltacortril and Precortisyl Forte.

The side effects of steroids taken at high doses for prolonged periods (oral steroids) can include: high blood sugar/diabetes, hunger, cataracts, glaucoma, psychiatric disturbances, stomach ulcers, the increased likelihood of infection, depression, sleeplessness, aggravation of schizo-phrenia and epilepsy, suppression of the adrenal glands, thin bones (osteoporosis), roundness of the face, high blood pressure, retarded growth in children, thinning of the skin (looking like stretch marks), excessive hair growth especially for females or a general feeling of being unwell.

To help counter some of the side effects of steroids take a mineral supplement which is high in calcium and Vitamin D and exercise regularly.

Combination of reliever and preventer medication

A combination of drugs containing both reliever and preventer medication is becoming more commonly prescribed. Possible side effects from combination drugs are similar to those from long-acting and preventer medication taken together. The drug and brand names are: Budesonide and Formoterol commonly known as Symbicort and Fluticasone and Salmeterol commonly known as Seretide.

New developments with anti-inflammatory medication

A new class of preventer anti-inflammatory drugs commonly known as Singulair came on the market in the 1990s. The main action of these drugs is to inhibit the powerful effects of inflammatory mediators called Leukotrienes. They work differently to steroids and it will be some time before the true effects become known. History has been unfavourable to drugs for the treatment of asthma and often it is ten or twenty years before the side effects become known.

Singulair comes in five and ten mg tablets and the side effects can include: fever, respiratory infection, stomach upset, dry mouth, weakness, dizziness, severe allergic reaction, headache, sleeplessness and muscle or joint pain.

It is not advised that these tablets are taken by children under six years of age or by patients with Churg-Strauss syndrome.

Other medication

Listed above are only the most commonly prescribed drugs for the treatment of asthma; there are other drugs used as preventers such as Sodium Cromoglycate (Intal for children or Tilade for adults), anticholinergics and bronchodilators known as Xantines. Xantines tend to be used less frequently now due to the many side effects connected with them.

Buteyko Clinic Method and medication

While it is not known exactly how steroids work, it is accepted that they treat inflammation which is the underlying airway obstruction.[6] Professor Buteyko regards steroids as the treatment of choice. His belief is that steroids work by reducing breathing and this occurs as quickly as one hour after being taken (oral). By reducing the breathing, airways are opened without a further loss of carbon dioxide. Professor Buteyko believes that taking the correct dosage of steroids is fundamental to maintaining safe control but unfortunately many people do not take the correct dose. Some people take too low a dose with the result that the asthma is uncontrolled and the risk of a severe attack remains present. Alternatively, some people start with a too-high dose that is not tapered downwards in accordance with the improvement in their condition. The British *Guidelines on Asthma Management*[7] advocates that 'there is evidence that all of the inhaled steroids are absorbed to some extent from the lung and hence will have some systemic activity. It is prudent therefore, as with all treatment, to give the lowest dose of inhaled steroid compatible with asthma control'. It is also advised to step down the dosage of steroids once the asthma is under control, although the *Guidelines* recognises that this 'is often not implemented'. Any reduction in steroid intake should be slow and only in conjunction with your doctor because patients respond at different rates when their doses are tapered.

Other patients rely too heavily on reliever medication and are fearful of steroid medication. Patients who rely predominantly on large doses of reliever medication for many years will have continuous symptoms and feel debilitated. Reliever medication can also pose a risk to a person's health and life. The management of asthma has changed over the years and people no longer need to rely on large amounts of reliever medication for their treatment.

Long-acting reliever inhalers which have become popular in recent years are very powerful and are taken at regular intervals regardless of whether they are needed or not. In addition, it has been reported that tolerance to long-acting bronchodilators may develop, meaning that the effect of the drug, especially when used as the mainstay of treatment, diminishes with constant use. Intermittent use would therefore be preferable.[8]

The ingredients of long-acting reliever inhalers are also present in a number of combination inhalers. For example the brand name Seretide is a combination of Serevent (long-acting reliever) and Flixotide (preventer).

Buteyko's view is that regular intake of bronchodilator medicine via inhaler or nebuliser overrides the body's defence mechanism. When the airways are forced open by bronchodilating drugs, hyperventilation is increased and the body will activate an even greater defence to prevent the further loss of CO_2. This leads to deterioration with a greater amount of reliever medication necessary to maintain control and, for this reason, it is important that the amount of reliever medication taken is minimal. History has proved his view to be correct and now the death rate has begun to decline as the treatment of choice has switched from relieving the sufferer to a more preventative approach.

History of medication

In 1949, a scientist called Hench and his team developed synthetic cortisone, which mimics the body's own naturally produced steroid. They were later awarded the Nobel Prize for Medicine for their achievements. Although steroids were introduced in the 1950s, there was very little known about what the correct dosage should be. As a result, large doses were prescribed resulting in many side effects. As soon as patients came off steroids, they suffered relapses and so required long-term treatment for control of asthma.

The serious side effects caused medical professionals to switch to bronchodilator reliever drugs as the favoured treatment for asthma. Reliever medication has a very powerful, quick acting effect, relaxing muscles to force the airways open. One puff of a short-acting reliever, such as Ventolin, will bring relief for three to four hours. The premise was that by taking a reliever on a regular basis, control could be maintained over the long term. However, over time, it was realised that this too may not be the best approach.

The relationship between an increase in the death rate and the increased use of reliever medication has been well documented. For example, deaths in Britain rose from 1,500 a year to 2,000 a year while prescriptions for reliever medication increased from eight million to 15 million.[9] In New Zealand an epidemic of asthma deaths occurred during the '70s and '80s believed to be caused by the reliever drug Fenoterol. Studies concluded that patients who used Fenoterol had a far greater chance of suffering a fatal asthma attack than those who didn't.[10,11,12,13] While this drug has been banned in New Zealand, it is still prescribed in Britain.

Overuse can be classified as taking more than three puffs of Ventolin per day. If this is the case then reduced breathing should be applied intensively. If it is not proving possible to reduce the need for reliever medication to three puffs within a short time, then preventer medication is necessary for a short period.

Taking a large quantity of reliever inhaler every day leads to increased tolerance to the medication.[14] There is a great risk with this, as the reliever eventually may not work in an emergency situation.[15,16] Overuse of reliever medication has been described as putting paint on rust; the symptoms are suppressed while the underlying condition gets progressively worse. The body fights back because the protective mechanism is removed by the reliever. This results in greater difficulty maintaining control and increases the risk of a serious attack.

Regular use of short-acting reliever inhalers leads to increased exercise induced bronchoconstriction.[17] This is not particularly well known among many sports coaches who always recommend taking reliever medication before exercise. The continuous use of reliever medication will in the long term exacerbate exercise-induced asthma. If reliever medication is required before exercise it begins to cause chronic hyperventilation and therefore the likelihood of having an attack during exercise is high. It would be far safer to refrain from competitive sport until the control pause is high and it is possible to participate in exercise without the need to take the inhaler beforehand. Alternatively an exercise such as walking that does not require advance reliever medication should be chosen. See the section on sport for how to prevent an asthma attack during exercise.

Towards the late '80s, the emphasis switched back to using steroids but this time in far smaller doses administered by inhaler; reliever medication was to be taken only when needed.

This change has reduced the death rate and highlights that it takes many years of trial and error before medical drugs are introduced and before the effects of them are fully known. When drugs are initially tested, it is for a relatively short period of time and just on a small sample of the population, maybe one or two thousand.

Since the 1990s there has been a decrease in the death rate directly as a result of introducing steroid inhalers. Steroids can cause side effects when taken in large quantities and over a long period of time. However, the quantities involved in inhaled steroids are too low to generate concern.

Some people are very hesitant of taking steroids partly because of the mistakes made in the '60s and partly because of the misconception that they may be anabolic steroids. However, if you require inhaled steroid, the risk from not taking it is far greater than from taking it. Reliance on reliever medication causes irreversible damage to the airways and increases the risk of serious and fatal attack. Once admitted to hospital, the amount of steroids administered would be a lot greater, so it makes more sense to manage asthma with a small quantity of inhaled steroid in the long term to avoid this risk.

The human body produces natural steroids in the adrenal cortex located on the outer surface of the adrenal gland. Without this natural steroid, the body would cease to function. It is believed by Professor Buteyko that hyperventilation causes the adrenals to produce fewer steroids than what is required by the body. As a result there is a need to supplement the difference between what the body produces and what is required with synthetic steroids. While the direct relationship between hyperventilation and inflammation may never be proven, scientific trials have demonstrated a reduction in the need for steroids when hyperventilation is reduced. For example, the volume of breath per minute of the Buteyko group at the trials at the Mater Hospital, Brisbane, was 14.1 litres. After three months, this had reduced to an average of 9.6 litres and the need for steroids had reduced by forty-nine per cent.

Since the mid 1990s long-acting bronchodilators and combination inhalers containing this medication have become very popular. Common long-acting bronchodilators are traded under the brand names of Serevent, Oxis, Spireva and Foradil. On January 23rd, 2003 the Food and Drug Administration (FDA) in the US announced: 'The drug [Serevent] may be associated with an increased risk of life-threatening asthma episodes or asthma related deaths, particularly in some patients.'[18] Then, on August 14th, 2003 the Reuters newsagency headline read: 'New warnings added to Glaxo Asthma Drugs' and the report declared that 'Serevent and Advair will carry new warnings about a higher, though small, risk of life-threatening asthma attacks and deaths, U.S. regulators said.'

chapter 9

how to help children and teenagers

'To know even one life has breathed easier because you have lived. This is to have succeeded.'

— Ralph Waldo Emerson (1803–1882)

This chapter contains breathing exercises and information that can be taught to children. Parents are advised not to rely solely on this chapter but to read the entire book in order to understand the whole concept of reduced breathing. It is recommended that this chapter is used for revision purposes only. For parents, working with their own asthmatic children to correct their breathing can be a challenge, but three case studies appended at the end of this chapter prove that it is a challenge worth the effort.

There are five steps that must be taken to correct a child's breathing, each of which will be explored in greater detail. The steps are: unblocking the nose, switching from mouth to nasal breathing, knowing what causes asthma, learning to relax the body and learning exercises to reduce the volume of air inhaled.

Unblocking the nose

A child's nose becomes blocked mainly due to overbreathing. Nasal passages constrict and mucus secretion increases, narrowing the space through which the child breathes. It feels like not enough air is passing through the nose and as a result the child will switch to mouth breathing. This creates a vicious circle because an even greater amount of carbon dioxide is lost. This increased loss of carbon dioxide causes the nasal passages to constrict even further and so the child continues to mouth breathe, possibly for the rest of his or her life. The most important factor in correcting breathing is learning to unblock the nose, a very simple and effective exercise.

The nose unblocking exercise involves holding the breath to temporarily increase carbon dioxide levels in the blood. The increase of carbon dioxide will then open the nasal passages within five minutes.

To perform this exercise, again using our hypothetical little girl called Emily as our example, she should sit down with her back straight, take a small breath in (two seconds) through the nose if possible and a small breath out (three seconds). If she is unable to take a breath in through the nose, a tiny breath in should be taken through the corner of the mouth. The child should then hold her nose with her fingers to stop the air flow and nod her head gently or sway her body until she cannot hold her breath any longer. It is important that Emily holds her nose until she feels a relatively strong need to breathe in.

Once Emily experiences the need to breathe in, she may let go of her nose and breathe gently through it, keeping the

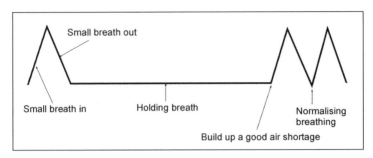

How to unblock the nose naturally

mouth closed. Sometimes Emily will take a breath in through the mouth when she lets go of her nose. At other times, she may open her mouth during the exercise. In both situations explain that she should keep her mouth closed. Practise the exercises with her until she is able to do it correctly.

Parents should supervise their child during the exercise and immediately afterwards should listen to the child's breathing and encourage her to reduce it to retain the increased level of carbon dioxide. The child should continue to do this exercise until the nose is unblocked. If it does not totally unblock, wait for about two minutes and perform the exercise again. It may be necessary to practise five or six times until the nose is unblocked.

Holding the breath traps additional carbon dioxide that has been produced from moving the head or swaying the body. At the start, it is common practice for the child's nose to become blocked again shortly after doing this exercise. This is because Emily's underlying breathing has not been changed and the body has not become accustomed to the increased carbon dioxide. After some time and with regular practise of breathing exercises, the child's body will become accustomed to a higher level of carbon dioxide and the nose will remain unblocked.

If the child is having difficulty unblocking her nose while shaking her head, then she should perform *Steps*, a process which will be explained later on.

The nose sounds the first warning call when overbreathing occurs by becoming the first part of the respiratory system to constrict. As soon as a child's nose starts to become blocked they should be assisted to unblock it with the nose unblocking exercise or with *Steps*.

Switching from mouth to nose breathing

It is important that all children breathe solely through the nose. Children can be helped to understand the importance of breathing through the nose by having the following points explained to them.

The air that we breathe in is not totally clean. It contains a large amount of dirt including germs, smoke and other filthy particles even though we may not be able to see it. The nose contains tiny cleaners, which cleanse this air before it goes into the body. If the air sneaks in through the mouth, dirty air is being sucked in which can make asthma worse, resulting in coughing or wheezing.

Air that sneaks in through the mouth is cold and dry while air that comes in through the nose is warm and moist and is better for the body. Ask the child if she would rather be warm (but not too warm) or very cold. Most will answer that they would rather be warm, so tell them that the inside of the body also likes air to be warm but this only happens by breathing through the nose.

Tell the child that by opening the mouth and breathing through it asthma will enter and slowly eat away at the inside of the body, especially at the airways. The more breathing through the mouth takes place, the more bronchial asthma will nibble at the airways and this will cause an attack. By breathing through the nose, bronchial asthma gets caught in the channels and by the tiny hairs that are in the centre of

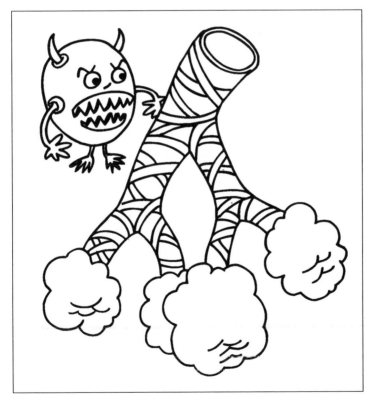

Asthma eating the airways

the nose. This prevents bronchial asthma from getting into the body to nibble at the lungs.

Finally, check that the child is aware of why she should breathe through the nose and help her to understand how important this really is. Reinforce the importance of breathing through the nose all of the time.

Breathing through the mouth is a bad habit and is common among children with asthma. For the first few weeks of the exercises the child will alternate between mouth breathing and nasal breathing. To make the switch to nasal breathing permanent, parents must play a significant role in observing the child's breathing and in telling the child when she is breathing through her mouth. This does entail a certain amount of persistence and observation from parents but it will reap untold health benefits for the child. The length of time it takes for the child to make a permanent switch to nasal breathing is dependent on the observations of parents and the attention the child pays to breathing.

If a very young child experiences difficulty learning to breathe through the nose, then it may be helpful for them to suck a dummy. This will cause the mouth to close, which will encourage nose breathing. Although some reports suggest that sucking a dummy is bad for a child's teeth, these reports are inconclusive. On the other hand, children who mouth breathe have far poorer health and a much higher number of cavities and incidence of gum disease than children who breathe through the nose.[1]

Knowing what causes asthma

It is important that children understand that big breathing causes asthma. The best way to explain big breathing is by blowing air onto a child's finger. At first blow a large amount of air – with a big, noisy puff – onto the finger and explain to her that this is big breathing. Then breathe a tiny amount of air onto the finger and explain that correct breathing means a small amount of air with almost nothing felt on the finger.

Big breathing is the cause of asthma and to make it easy for the child to understand explain that Emily is big breathing if she is breathing with her mouth.

By getting the child to repeat this explanation of what causes her asthma, parents can determine whether Emily understands the relationship between big breathing and her symptoms. Once the child understands and can tell others the difference between big breathing and correct breathing, she can proceed to the next level which is reducing the volume of air inhaled.

Learning to relax the body

It is important that the child remains relaxed throughout the day and especially before, during and after breathing exercises. Tension increases the rate of breathing because it results in a reduced blood flow and a consequent reduction in the amount of oxygen reaching tissues and organs. A child's asthma symptoms are generally worse following a period of anger, emotion or tension.

To explain relaxation, tell the child to think of jelly on a plate and ask this question: what would the jelly do if the plate was carried across the room? Children usually say that the jelly wobbles but if your child is not sure, explain that jelly is normally soft and wobbly. Make some jelly for tea if you have to! Make it clear that when we are relaxed we are all soft and wobbly too, just like jelly on a plate.

Demonstrate how to become soft and wobbly by standing up and letting your shoulders fall to the resting position, allowing your arms and body to go soft and limp. Become floppy and sway your body gently and ask your child to copy you. Remember, this is supposed to be fun, and your child will enjoy watching you 'messing'. Explain that this is relaxation and that when we are relaxed, we breathe less and as a result asthma attacks are reduced.

There is a very simple test that can be applied to determine whether a child like our Emily is relaxed. Lift up her

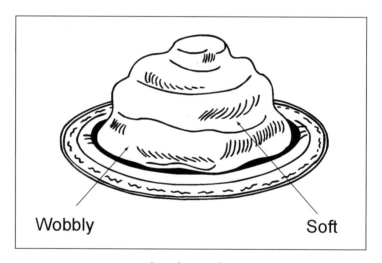

Wobbly   Soft

Learning to relax

arm; if it is heavy she is relaxed, if it is light the child is helping you to raise her arm. Ask her to become floppy and wobbly like jelly and her arm should become heavy on lifting.

Exercises to reduce the volume of air inhaled

Once Emily has a good understanding of nasal breathing, big breathing and relaxation, she can proceed to the next level of reduced breathing using special exercises. The primary exercise for children is called *Steps* and *Mouse Breathing* is the secondary exercise. *Mouse Breathing* is the name used to describe the process of reduced breathing in children.

The steps exercise helps children to make great progress with their breathing and is also helpful as a measurement of progress if a child is unable to apply the control pause. *Steps* involves physical activity which will increase carbon dioxide combined with holding the breath which will trap this carbon dioxide.

To perform *Steps*, children should practise the following. Tell them to take a small breath in (two seconds) followed by a small breath out (three seconds). They should then hold the breath by pinching the nose. It is better if the child holds her nose by raising her hand above the mouth so that the mouth remains visible. This way, if a child like Emily takes a breath in through the mouth, it will be noticeable.

Encourage her to walk as many steps as she can until she needs to breathe in again. Count aloud every five or ten steps to motivate the child to take as many steps as possible.

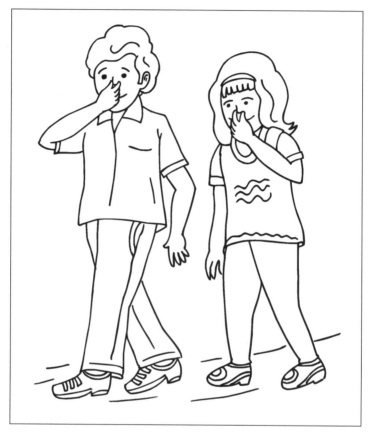

Doing *Steps*

When the child recommences breathing, it must be only through the nose and breathing must be calmed immediately. If the child's shoulders rise and become tense, point it out and ask her to let her shoulders drop to the resting position.

Usually the first breath after completing *Steps* will be bigger than normal. Make sure the child then reduces or suppresses the second and third breaths. It is important that

Emily relaxes and becomes as soft as jelly because the more she relaxes, the quicker the recovery of breathing will be.

Count each step aloud and record the number so that progress can be evaluated and compare each day's steps with the previous few days. *Steps* can be used as a measurement tool if the child is unable to do the control pause correctly, and she should be encouraged to increase the number of steps she takes over time. The goal is for children to be able to walk a hundred steps without having to take a breath. This might sound like a tough standard but it is very feasible. *Steps* should be done walking but not running, but fast walking is fine.

If Emily becomes stressed or pushes too hard, it will take a number of breaths to calm her breathing. When this occurs, reduce the number of steps that she takes.

Steps can be interspersed with reduced breathing called *Mouse Breathing* and the sequence this should follow is explained later in this chapter.

This exercise requires concentration in order to be practised correctly so the child should be taken to a quiet place where there will be no distractions. With this exercise the child sits down, adopts the correct posture with the back straight and the head looking forward.

Emily should be encouraged to relax her shoulders, allowing them to fall to their natural position. Raised or tense shoulders increase the volume of the chest cavity and so increase the volume of air that is inhaled. Tension increases breathing while relaxation decreases breathing. Therefore it's especially important to relax the muscles involved in respiration.

The child should place a finger under the nose in a horizontal position so that the air flowing through the nostrils can be monitored. The finger should be placed just above the top lip, close enough to the nostrils to feel the air flow, but not so close that the flow will be blocked.

Encourage the child to pretend that she is a little white mouse and that there is a big hungry cat waiting outside the door listening for any sound that the mouse makes. Explain that the cat has excellent hearing and will know that there is a mouse present if it hears the mouse breathing. The child

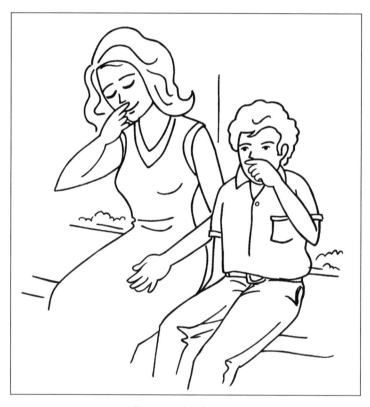

Finger under the nose

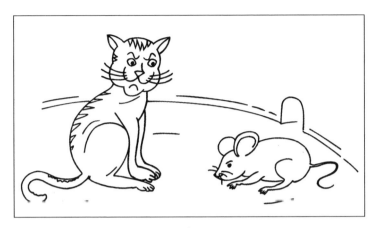

Cat and mouse

will instinctively reduce her breathing to avoid being captured by the cat.

The aim of this exercise is to reduce the volume of air exhaled onto the finger. The greater the amount of warm air felt on the out breath, the greater breathing is. Encourage the child to concentrate on reducing the amount of warm air felt on the finger.

With this exercise, when the depth of breathing is reduced, the breathing rate (number of breaths taken per minute) may increase. This is completely normal. Do not be concerned with the number of breaths per minute as this will change according to the volume and the aim is to reduce this volume.

The aim of all breathing exercises is to condition the body to accept a higher level of carbon dioxide. There are two main ways to do this: by reducing the breathing by monitoring the air-flow with mouse breathing and by reducing breathing through physical activity, *Steps* and outdoor exercise.

Exercises are best performed in blocks of twenty minutes, two to three times per day. Spending less time than this only temporarily increases the carbon dioxide.

A commonly practised sequence of exercises for most children is detailed below and exercise sheets especially for children to record the amount of steps are included at the back of this book.

Exercises should be completed in the order set out below, with intermittent breaks.

CP	Steps	Steps	Steps	CP	Steps	Steps	Steps	Mouse Breathing 3-5 min.	CP

A relatively smooth session with no breaks will take about twenty minutes. This should be practised twice a day for two to three months, preferably before breakfast and before dinner. All exercises are better practised before meals as food intake decreases the number of steps that can be taken and may lead to cramps. Times do not have to be exact but should be as close as possible to those set out above.

A rest should also be taken after every set of exercises in order to avoid overdoing them as this can result in a headache. If a child does experience distress, then stop the exercises and concentrate on relaxation. Exercises can be resumed later that day or the following day with special observation on applying the correct intensity of exercises.

A rest is taken before each control pause to ensure it is measured accurately. A control pause that is taken directly after reduced breathing will be lower than after a rest. If the child is unable to perform a CP or reduced breathing then replace both with an extra set of *Steps*. (*Steps* can be also used as a measurement of progress.) Every two steps constitutes one second of the control pause. When the child is able to perform a hundred steps, her control pause is estimated to be fifty seconds. In practice, a child may be able to perform a hundred steps but may only have a control pause of twenty seconds. In this situation, *Steps* is the more accurate guide of progress.

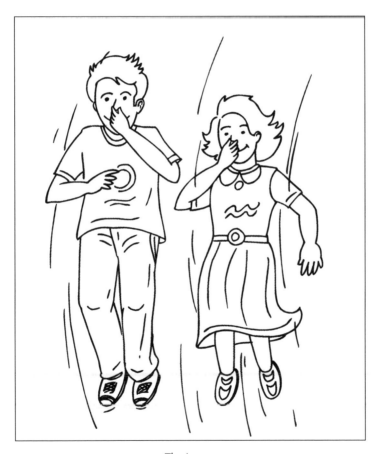

The Jumps

Everyone knows children can have a short attention span so if the child becomes bored with doing exercises, then *Steps* can be replaced with breath-holding while playing hopscotch, squats, jumping jacks or swimming (in the case of swimming, aim to increase the amount of strokes or time spent under water between each breath).

Remember, the aim of these exercises is to eliminate asthma symptoms by switching to nasal breathing and normalising the carbon dioxide levels. This should always be kept in mind when practising exercises and monitoring the progress which has been made.

How to stop an asthma attack

If a child is experiencing difficulty breathing, it is better to refrain from doing *Steps* as it can cause a large inhalation on completion, which can exacerbate an attack. In this instance it is safer for the child to perform *Mouse Breathing* to control the asthma attack and to continue with *Steps* only when her breathing has calmed.

As soon as the first signs of an attack appear – a blocked nose, wheezing, coughing or tightening of the airways – the child should practise the exercise below. If the child is un-able to obtain relief within five minutes, then her reliever medication should be administered. If she experiences a severe attack, medication should be given or medical assis-tance sought immediately.

However, the following exercise can prove very effective in stopping an attack when applied during the early stages.

Sit the child in an upright position. If Emily is lying down in bed make her get up and sit instead. If the room is stuffy, open the window to let in fresh air.

At the first signs of an attack, encourage the child to resist the urge to take big breaths. It is important to focus on remaining calm and it may also help to have Emily repeat to herself, over and over again, the words 'relax and remain calm'.

It is important that Emily does not reduce her breathing too much as this may lead to an increase in breathing which will exacerbate the attack.

An asthma attack can be a frightening experience and a child will naturally become tense as anxiety and panic set in. The struggle to breathe can also create both mental and emotional stress and a vicious circle is activated because the asthma attack increases stress levels which in turn leads to increased hyperventilation.

A very useful exercise as a parent is to gently massage the shoulders of the child. This is not difficult to accomplish and anyone can do it. Gentle pressure should be applied by massaging the muscles located in the chest, shoulder and neck region while repeating the words 'relax and breathe less' to the child.

Increased tension brought about by the attack will only result in making it worse. A massage can offer comfort to a child because it has a very calming and reassuring effect, helping Emily to come out of the discomfort being experienced as a result of the asthma attack.

This might be construed as a provocative statement but, in some cases, children have been known to start an asthma attack in order to get attention from their parents. They subconsciously know that their tantrum or anger will cause deep breathing and lead to an attack. It is important to remember that an asthma attack is always serious regardless of how it started. At the first signs of an attack – a blocked nose – help the child to breathe like a little mouse and to perform *nose unblocking exercise*. If the attack is not under control within a few minutes, then whatever medication has been prescribed should be taken. Don't prolong the attack or have your child experience unnecessary discomfort by delaying the taking of reliever medication. After she has taken this medication, ask her to remain as soft as jelly and to breathe as gently as possible. If reliever medication is not working correctly within five to ten minutes, seek medical attention immediately.

Parents' behaviour during an asthma attack

An asthma attack can be best compared to trying to breathe while a pillow is pressed down on your face. This greatly restricts breathing and creates anxiety, stress, uncertainty, fear and panic, especially for a child. If a child is suffering an asthma attack sit her down and help her to relax in a cool environment.

As parents, try not to be visibly upset, to cry or to panic in front of the child. This can be a very difficult thing to do but remaining calm will help reduce the anxiety being experienced by the child. Instilling a sense of fear and panic in the child will exacerbate the attack and can cause a lot of harm. Likewise, do not encourage the child to pay too much attention to their condition. Repeating phrases like 'poor David has asthma' or 'you're so unfortunate to have asthma' leads to the child thinking negatively about her own condition and will result in a deterioration of the child's asthma in the long term.

On a more positive note, parents often experience great peace of mind when they begin to observe an improvement in their child's condition using the exercises outlined and when the child realizes that it's possible to have some control over her condition. This will lead to the parents offering greater encouragement to the child to continue with the breathing exercises and to implement other lifestyle changes.

Knowing what causes asthma

People often have a number of questions about asthma and one of those most frequently asked is this: how does a baby develop asthma when many of the conditions responsible for causing overbreathing do not apply?

Children often develop asthma at a very early age, in some cases as young as three months old. Professor Buteyko believes that deep breathing exercises taught to expectant mothers during pregnancy is the main contributory factor. The deep breathing carried out by the expectant mother lowers the levels of carbon dioxide in her body and this, in turn, lowers the level of carbon dioxide for her embryo.

When the baby is born, he or she may receive a slap on the bottom, causing the baby to start breathing with a deep first breath. A life of overbreathing begins at that crucial first moment of life. Although it has not been proved that excessive breathing by mothers may be passed to the child, it is a theory that does merit consideration.

It is a mother's instinct to protect her newborn baby and it is quite common, due to good intentions, to ensure a baby is kept excessively warm. Some mothers have even recalled beads of sweat on their baby's forehead as a result of their efforts to keep them warm on a cold Winter night. The truth is that babies have a very high metabolism, which generates much more energy than an adult and means they can tolerate cooler temperatures. A practice performed by a number of older nurses involves stripping children naked and leaving them for a number of hours lying without any covers. In this situation the nurse understands the benefits of a cool environment to the child, even though he or she may not know exactly why. Very warm temperatures and excess synthetic clothing increase breathing while cool temperatures reduce it.

It is also interesting to note that babies who are breast fed for at least the first four months of life are substantially less likely to develop asthma than those who are fed on milk formulas.[2,3,4,5]

Formula is processed and can also contain traces of aluminium from the can. It is not an ideal substitute for the milk that nature intended babies to drink. Breast milk has been refined by nature throughout evolution and contains the perfect mix of protein and nutrients for the healthy development of a newborn. Increased protein levels and traces of aluminium (which are toxic) will lead to an increase in breathing. Many parents have observed the onset of asthma and eczema in their child soon after making the switch from breast milk to mass-produced processed formulas.

Parents' behaviour

It has often been observed at clinics that a child's breathing exactly mirrors that of the parents. Both respiratory rates and other traits, such as sighing, can function in synchronisation. Without doubt, the breathing of parents in part influences the overbreathing of a child.

If the child's father walks around the house with his mouth open puffing and panting and being unobservant of his breathing, then the child will do likewise. Often, it is the behaviour of parents that slows down the progress of children. Correct breathing is a family affair and it is beneficial for the health of all family members, even if they do not have asthma. Teaching the child to do one thing while everyone else in the family continues with their bad habits and unhealthy lifestyles will not help the child. Children learn best through example. This is very important for parents who wish to help a child with asthma. In fact, the child is unlikely to make progress unless the parents also adopt reduced breathing as a way of life.

Another negative influence on the child's progress can be the attitude of the parents. On commencing breathing exercises, it is important that both parents display a positive attitude towards correcting the child's breathing. The simple fact is that unless a child receives encouragement to adopt nasal breathing and practise *Steps*, the child will not understand the importance of breathing correctly and as a result will not pay any attention to it. A sceptical parent would be far better off keeping their opinions quiet rather than making negative comments about breath retraining. The child's progress within just a number of weeks will be enough to discount their initial scepticism.

In order to be aware of a child's breathing pattern it is important to understand what factors may cause a child to overbreathe and these factors should then be eliminated. Parents should monitor a child's condition by observation and by measuring their CP during the day and after various activities (if the child is unable to understand the concept of reduced breathing, then measure the number of steps they can walk).

This detective work will provide some insight into what is causing the overbreathing and therefore the symptoms. Many children become so focused on certain activities that they are completely oblivious of the fact that their mouths are open or that they are big breathing. It takes time for a child to make the switch but when she does, mouth breathing will feel peculiar and strange and she will naturally revert to nasal breathing.

While the child is outdoors, there may be times when there is a quantity of dust, exhaust fumes from cars or any other agent in the air. To avoid inhaling these particles, the child should be told that if they ever see or smell dirty air, she should hold her breath and walk away. If she is unable to walk away, encourage her to reduce their breathing. Both of these practices will greatly reduce the amount of dirty air that enters the airways.

Children should be encouraged to play outside and to do as much physical activity as possible while they are out in the fresh air. If a child is symptomatic, then physical activity is not encouraged because it will lead to overbreathing. Years ago, children played outdoors, ate less generally and not nearly the amount of junk food eaten today. Houses were cooler and fresh air often ran throughout them in the form of draughts. It can be argued that children were much healthier in those days; the incidence of asthma was certainly much lower.

Sequence of training

When teaching a child, a step-by-step approach is often best, enabling the child like our imaginary little girl, Emily, to move onto different levels as her knowledge improves. The following is a typical scenario of a young child commencing breath retraining.

The first week is spent teaching Emily the reasons why it is so important to breathe through the nose and the child is taught to use only this way of breathing for every event and situation. If the child is at school, then it is helpful to explain to the teacher exactly what is happening and ask them to be observant of Emily's breathing. At any time, if she is observed breathing through the mouth, then she should be reminded of the reasons why it is not good to breathe this way.

By positive reinforcement, it can be explained that asthma will improve dramatically with continued nasal breathing, or by negative reinforcement that dirty germs and filthy air will enter their airways and eat away at the lungs. The child should be asked at regular times throughout the day why is it so important to breathe through the nose and not through the mouth.

When Emily understands the importance of nasal breathing and breathes through the nose for most of the day and night, then it is onto the next stage of teaching, and *Steps* and the importance of being relaxed are introduced. Initially these are practised without the control pause and mouse breathing. *Steps* is to be practised two to three times each day. When the child is competent in doing *Steps*, the control pause and mouse breathing can be introduced.

If a child is having difficulty in applying exercises, training should not be abandoned. A softly, softly approach generally produces good results.

All children should be taught the importance of reduced breathing and breathing through the nose. Instead, the typical approach is to administer potent chemicals to the child often from a very early age. It is sad to hear of young children being treated with nebulisers and large doses of steroids on a regular basis. If these children had been taught how to breathe correctly, their symptoms and attacks would be greatly reduced or eliminated entirely. The amount of suffering and medication that each child would be exposed to therefore would be significantly less.

Relapse

It is common for children to experience a relapse in the first six months. This can be part of the cleansing reaction, as symptoms may get a little worse before they get better. During this reaction, a lot of mucus clears from the lower airways and can result in coughing or wheezing. At other times, the relapse is due to the child becoming relaxed about their breathing, missing steps or reverting to mouth breathing for a few days. When a relapse occurs and the child is wheezy or coughing, then do not do the *Steps* exercise as it can cause the child to take big breaths on completion. Instead, perform mouse breathing while having a medium air shortage. Generally, the relapse is for two to three days only and afterwards the child will continue where they left off in relation to their control pause, *Steps* and asthma.

It is always helpful to remember that the very factors that caused big breathing are still present. For example, if the child continues to eat a lot of junk food, drinks no pure water, performs no exercise and remains in very warm clothing or stuffy rooms, then big breathing will ensue.

Case studies

To demonstrate what can be achieved, case studies have been compiled on three children – Robert, Clara and Lorcan – who attended workshops with their parents. [These case studies have been compiled from conversations with the parents of the children and have been included with their permission. Surnames are not disclosed to protect their confidentiality.]

Robert

Robert is a five-year-old child from Mayo who first attended the Galway Asthma Care Clinic with his mother on March 25th, 2003. Robert had mild to moderate asthma requiring two to three puffs of Ventolin per day. In addition to his asthma, he had chronic tiredness, irritability, lack of energy and frequent headaches. He was taught the very basics of the programme and his mum was asked to participate in the observation and application of Robert's exercises.

Robert's task was to practise reduced breathing and *Steps* every day. Each month he was set the task of completing an extra ten steps. Soon he could do seventy steps quite easily and on a number of occasions reached one hundred. On follow up, his mother was overjoyed with the improvement in Robert's condition. Not only had his asthma improved so dramatically that he had no symptoms and no requirement for medication, but he also had far more energy and no headaches. He could now enjoy the same activities as other children his age.

Clara

Nine-year-old Clara lives in Dublin and was diagnosed with asthma at the age of four. On March 2nd, 2003, Clara attended an Asthma Care clinic accompanied by her mother and grandmother. Here is Clara's history prior to that date.

She did not suffer from wheezing or coughing. Her main problem was recurrent chest infections, which she often had on a monthly basis prior to March 2003. Each time, a course of antibiotics would be prescribed.

Consistently, Clara looked pale and had black bags under her eyes which is a typical feature of many asthmatics. Her peak flow reading averaged 250 and her personal best was 275. Her daily medication requirement was four puffs of Seretide 125 to control her wheezing and Nasocort for unblocking her nose. She took Ventolin as prescribed by her doctor whenever she had a chest infection.

Clara's grandmother, who looked after her for much of the day, was present at the clinic. She assisted Clara in her practice of steps each day and in applying other recommendations as part of the programme.

Here is a synopsis of her progress: March 2nd, eighteen steps; April 2nd, fifty steps; May 2nd, fifty-five steps; June 2nd, eighty steps and a CP of forty-two seconds; July 2nd, eighty-six steps and a CP of fifty-one seconds, and August 2nd, a CP of one minute and fifteen seconds.

Clara's doctor changed her medication from Seretide and reduced her dosage to two puffs of 125 mg Flixotide a day. She did experience a temporary relapse and had a chest infection during the first week of June. An antibiotic was required for this and three puffs of Ventolin were taken during one day.

She recovered from her chest infection quickly and her peak flow reverted to between 290 and 310. Her grandmother calls the clinic frequently to ask questions and also to report on her progress. Clara continues to make excellent progress in recovering from her asthma and also looks far better; she has a healthier colour, feels better and knows herself how well she is doing. For the month of July 2002, Clara had three courses of antibiotics. She did not require any during July 2003. At the time of writing (December 2003), Clara has had only one chest infection since March. Her peak flow readings now average 350 and her medication intake has been substantially decreased by her GP.

Lorcan

Lorcan is aged ten and from Dublin. Lorcan attended a workshop in October 2002. His condition was continuously moderate, requiring daily preventer and reliever medication. His intake was two puffs of Flixotide per day and Ventolin when needed. Even with this preventative dose, Lorcan was unable to enjoy many of the activities children of his age take for granted. His mum explained that not alone was he having difficulty playing football, but that even standing at the side of a football pitch to watch a game on a windy day would be enough to start an attack.

In addition to asthma, he also suffered regular headaches and occasional tummy upsets. These are common symptoms of hyperventilation and are often present in many people with asthma. However, most people don't relate one to the other.

Lorcan practised steps each day and also applied other aspects of the breathing programme. Shortly afterwards, he was able to play football with his local team. Over the course of six months, his doctor reduced his Flixotide intake.

Lorcan is now totally free from all medication and symptoms, and his mother says the peace of mind she enjoys from this improvement is wonderful. She reported that Lorcan had taken part in a sailing trip around the Cork coast. She said he did the same trip previously but was plagued with symptoms. The second time, he participated in this voyage totally free from symptoms and entirely free from the need for medication. He still carries his reliever inhaler as advised, and will continue to do so for a year or so in the unlikely event that he may require it.

Summary of breathing exercises for children

Reduced air flow

+ Set time aside to do exercise with no distractions.
+ Sit down and adopt the correct posture.
+ Relax and become as soft and wobbly as jelly. Ask the child to pretend she is very wobbly just like jelly on a plate.
+ Place a finger under the nose without blocking the air flow [*Mouse Breathing*].
+ Concentrate on reducing the amount of air flow that is blown onto the finger by monitoring the temperature of air flow onto the finger.
+ Reduce movement of chest and tummy.
+ Observe breathing throughout the day.

Summary of Steps

+ Take a small breath in (two seconds) and a small breath out (three seconds).

+ Hold the breath and walk as many steps as possible until there is a strong desire to breathe in again.
+ After completion of steps relax like jelly and breathe like a little mouse.
+ Count aloud each step and record the number so that progress can be monitored.

Significant points

Other important points to remember are: young children should only sleep on their tummies and never on their backs; children should never eat before going to bed; the amount of junk food eaten should be reduced and a healthy lifestyle encouraged; children should only eat when hungry, and excessive clothing and temperatures should be avoided. Playing outdoors in the fresh air as much as possible during the day is beneficial while breathing through the nose all day.

chapter 10

individual
and national goals

'Nature does not hurry, yet everything is accomplished.'

– Lao Tzu

Correct breathing volume is a holistic approach and is probably the single most positive influence you can have on your health during your lifetime. Bearing this in mind, it should be approached with good intent, discipline and determination.

Your over-riding goal is to reduce the volume of air that passes through your lungs to more correct physiological levels. You know you are achieving this when you begin to feel better and when your control pause is increasing.

The **two steps** necessary are:

✦ Increased observation of breathing. Breathing is a twenty-four hour activity, so it is important to observe it periodically throughout the day. Pay attention to your breathing and ask yourself if it is gentle, calm, regular, silent and as still as if you are not breathing, or if it's noisy, irregular, uneven, raspy and loud. If your breathing sounds like the latter, then it's time to take steps to change it.

Activities such as eating, sleeping, stress, and physical activity affect breathing. By increasing your own awareness, you will notice many factors which increase your breathing. This may be your tendency to eat a huge meal, your stress levels at work, or it may be any one of other features of modern civilisation. After an Asthma Care Clinic, each participant is amazed at how conscious he or she becomes of his or her breathing. This is a vital step in the right direction because an improvement can only be made with increased awareness and knowledge of breathing.

✦ It will require considerable attention to reverse a bad habit which you have been unintentionally and unwittingly practising for all your life. Regular practice of breathing exercises is necessary to retrain the body to accept a reduced and healthier volume of breathing. It also helps you understand what it means exactly to breathe in a calm, gentle and regular manner.

For the first couple of months it is important to set aside time to perform breathing exercises. The reason for this is that you will not make progress if all your exercises are completed while reading a book, watching TV or driving because your concentration will be divided between doing the exercises and whatever else you're doing at the time. However, following a number of months' practice, you will be entirely familiar with the concept of reduced breathing and so will be able to apply it in almost any place or situation.

What to expect

Everyone can expect a substantial improvement in their condition within a short period of time. Coughing, wheezing, breathlessness and disruptions during the night will decrease. This initial time-frame can vary from one day to a couple of weeks.

Over the first six months, you may experience a setback which can last for a couple of days. This can be due to a cleansing reaction or it may be simply the fact that all asthmatics have good days and bad days, depending on environmental conditions and exposure to triggers. During your setbacks, practice reduced breathing and continue to take your medication. Take your short-acting reliever medication as needed and don't put yourself through any distress.

After your setback, your control pause will revert back to what it was before the attack. If the setback is due to a cleansing reaction, your control pause will increase from the level it was at before the attack.

As an example, the following is a typical scenario. You have been practising reduced breathing for two months and you have achieved a control pause of twenty seconds. During the third month, you experience a setback. Your control pause reverts to ten seconds for two days. You continue to practice reduced breathing during your setback. After the two days have passed, your control pause increases to twenty-two seconds.

This pattern will continue for some time. You can expect a steady improvement with reduced symptoms, interspersed some good days and some bad days. As time goes on, the number and severity of bad days will decline, and your symptoms will have reduced dramatically.

When your control pause reaches twenty seconds, you may reach a plateau and find that it's difficult to increase it. After a period of time, depending on the severity of your asthma and your commitment to reducing your breathing, your control pause will pass beyond twenty seconds.

Personally, I made my best progress using physical activity and I believe that no person with asthma can make very much progress without it. For the first few weeks of practising breathing exercises, it is better to avoid intense physical activity, especially if you require a reliever inhaler first.

The older you are, the more time you should spend exercising but at a less intensive level. Ideally, an older person should commit himself or herself to walking for one hour a day while breathing through the nose. I remember once talking to an acquaintance who told me his mother was aged ninety-seven. Out of curiosity, I asked him what was her secret for long life.

'Well,' he replied. 'Mam never smoked or drank; she always ate a small amount of food, mainly vegetables, and each day she walks from the house into town and back, a distance of about two miles.'

When your control pause reaches forty seconds, the amount of time you spend on exercises can be cut. By this time, carbon dioxide will be restored to the correct level and you will automatically breathe a healthier volume of air. Remember that under normal circumstances it is the level of carbon dioxide that determines your breathing and not oxygen. Your respiratory centre stimulates or relaxes breathing to maintain carbon dioxide at set levels. When carbon dioxide is set at a higher level, the volume of breathing will be calm, gentle and correct, to maintain this level. At this time, you will observe your breathing unconsciously, regardless of any activity you partake in. If you notice your breathing increasing at any time, you will also know how to reduce it.

Always remember that the factors that cause us to big breathe in the first place are still present in any modern society, and that it may not be possible to eliminate them entirely. We will continue to socialise, eat meat, drink alcohol, talk excessively, walk into stuffy environments and endure stress, for example.

However, because you will be more aware of your breathing and the effect that any of these triggers may have on you personally, their influence will be far less than before. Nevertheless, it is always beneficial to keep them in mind. If you allow your lifestyle to revert to drinking ten cups of coffee a day, eating a diet of processed food, doing no physical exercise and sleeping with your mouth open, then it will not be long before your carbon dioxide levels fall and your asthma symptoms return.

Why does breath correction not work for everyone?

Correction of breathing has a success rate of ninety per cent. This is a remarkably high figure considering that it is totally based on patient application. No therapy ever has a success rate of one hundred per cent, not even the most successful of medications.

There are three reasons why breath correction doesn't work for the other ten per cent of those who try it: laziness, a view that they don't have enough time for the exercises, and chronic focal infections which will naturally hamper progress.

Laziness

The most common reason some people give for neglecting to observe their breathing and practise their exercises is simply laziness. Breath retraining does require discipline and determination to reverse a life time of bad breathing, especially for the first few weeks.

Every now and then, a person – we'll call him John – will arrive into our clinic having been taught the importance of nasal breathing and reducing the volume of air inhaled. John will enter the room a week later with his mouth wide open and walk to his seat totally oblivious of his breathing. Panting, he will then sit down and make no attempt to control his breathing or to switch to nasal breathing. Luckily, this is only a rarity but at the same time, it is completely unnecessary.

Whenever I see this occurring, I find it disheartening. I always bring it to John's attention and try to reinforce the necessity of reducing overbreathing or at the very least, keeping the mouth closed. In this situation, it is almost guaranteed that John devoted no time to observing his breathing or doing his exercises, primarily from laziness.

Time constraints

Some people feel they don't have the time to invest an hour in their health each day. Like any good investment, you forsake now what you can reap later. An investment in your health surpasses any other, regardless of the monetary returns. If you think time is a problem, then you have two options. The first is to practise breathing exercises for a maximum of ninety minutes each day for three months. This is a total investment of 135 hours in your health.

Scientific trials in the Buteyko Method carried out at the Mater Hospital in Brisbane, Australia, concluded that there was a seventy per cent improvement in the condition; ninety per cent less need for reliever medication, and forty-nine per cent less need for steroids after three months. The results of a more recent trial at Gisborne Hospital, New Zealand were consistant with earlier findings. Upon reaching a control pause of forty seconds, momentary attention is all that is required to maintain an asthma-free life.

The second option is the one you are currently taking, the one that doesn't involve a small investment of 135 hours of your time in your health. If you are following this option, your breathing will probably increase as you get older, resulting in a deterioration of your asthma. The amount of medications that you will require will steadily increase. Not only will your medication intake increase but the strength will as well.

Cumulative side effects will start to become obvious after so many years' use of steroids and bronchodilators. Your skin may become weak and may break at the slightest touch; calcium may leak from your bones resulting in osteoporosis; you may start to gain weight, and diabetes may develop. If you are female you may grow hair on your body. These are just some of the possible side effects.

As you age and as your condition worsens, you will be prescribed a nebuliser and you may need to take this up to four times a day. On some days you may not be able to get up out of bed at all without taking it. Your quality of life will depend totally on your nebuliser and frequent use of medication. Over time, you will get wheezy and breathless at the slightest exertion, your nights will be disrupted on a regular basis, and your social life will be severely hampered.

This may be your life

That description of what lies ahead for many asthmatics and overbreathers is not intended to encourage you to stop taking medication. On the contrary, preventer steroidal medication is very necessary and death can result from failure to take it. The description of your possible future is included merely to illustrate the two options available to you. You might suggest that the second option never happens. Unfortunately it does. I have met far too many people in this situation. It is very real. This is not a scare tactic.

At each workshop, I often ask people to write down the following sentence: 'I get out of this exactly what I put in.' Remember, this therapy is not the quick fix. The quick fix is reaching for your reliever medication every time you experience symptoms.

Case studies

The following case studies are included to provide you with an insight into the effects of this therapy. I deliberately selected two severe chronic cases. I have not included the person's surname in either case to protect their identity.

Teresa

Sixty-one year old Dubliner Teresa attended an Asthma Care workshop on November 24th, 2002. She had been a chronic severe asthmatic for most of her life. Her normal maintenance dose of medication was 15 mg Deltacotril (oral steroids); two puffs of Seretide 500 each morning and evening, and Slophylum doses of 250 mg each morning and 500mg at night. She also took a Combivent nebuliser dose four times a day. In addition, she inhaled about five puffs of Ventolin per day. When Teresa suffered a relapse, her medication would be increased for a short period of time.

During the first day of the workshop, Teresa started to experience an attack of wheezing and coughing. I immediately instructed her to apply reduced breathing with a special breath hold exercise. After about two minutes, her symptoms decreased and she was able to carry on without having to take her reliever or nebuliser. This left Teresa in no doubt as to the effectiveness of reduced breathing exercises.

Over the weeks and months to follow, Teresa applied her reduced breathing programme diligently. She also took daily walks, observing her breathing during the physical activity. Within a short period of time, Teresa's symptoms reduced, allowing her to cut down on reliever medication. As the months passed, she visited her doctor on several occasions to have her medication intake reviewed. I remember speaking to her about six months later and her symptoms had improved considerably. At that time, she had no requirement for Ventolin or nebulisers and her maintenance dose of Deltacortril was reduced to 10mg per day. Her quality of life is now better than what it has been for many years and family and friends have told her that they have never seen her look better.

Marie

Seventy-one year old Dubliner Marie arrived at our Dublin workshop – in a wheelchair pushed by her son – on April 5th and 12th, 2003. Marie suffered from asthma and chronic obstructive pulmonary disease (COPD), a term used to describe patients with chronic bronchitis and emphysema. Marie was very debilitated. Her mobility was restricted because she didn't have 'enough breath' to get anywhere.

Our first step with Marie was to show her how to recognise her bad breathing and to bring considerable attention to nasal breathing. Exercises were tailored to meet her condition and to take into account her lack of mobility. Our main priority was to ensure that Marie made progress in a relaxed way. When someone suffers severe breathlessness, it is important that breathing exercises are not so stressful that they cause an increase in breathing. From the exercises provided, Marie made great progress and within a few weeks was able to leave the wheelchair to take small walks.

In this case, we applied walking as part of her program but ensured that she walked only as far as she could. If, for example, she felt she needed to take a breath in through the mouth, she stopped walking to give herself the chance to reduce and calm her breathing.

A number of months after Marie improved, I received a call from a woman enquiring about the workshop. She told me that Marie had given her the telephone number when the two women met in Spain. I thought about 'our' Marie and I couldn't help wondering if this woman's Spanish contact was the same Marie who had attended a workshop in a wheelchair. Shortly afterwards, I called 'our' Marie to see how she was getting on. She confirmed that she had been on holiday in Spain and – amazingly – had walked two miles each day she was there.

Marie said that when she returned to Ireland, she had a little difficulty walking two miles per day because the wind would trigger an attack. On hearing this, I suggested that she purchase a treadmill to use in the house. With the help of her children, she followed the suggestion and continues to use her treadmill to this day.

Most of us can walk two miles a day without much effort, so it may seem a small feat. However, for a person like Marie who had lost her mobility and who was totally dependent on her siblings and children, the ability to be able to do this again constitutes a tremendous improvement in quality of life. It is people like Marie who give me the impulse and drive to reach out to all people with the same condition.

On August 7th, 2003, Marie sent a letter to The Asthma Society of Ireland to tell them about her progress. She also sent me a copy of this letter which I reproduce here.

Dear X,

I am writing to you about the Buteyko Method. I am 71 years old and have COPD and asthma. I was wheelchair bound until last April and used a nebulizer five times a day. I could not go anywhere unless I was in a car or a wheelchair.

I saw a programme on Open House *about Buteyko. A friend found out for me. I went to the workshop on April 5th, 2003 and again on the 12th for four hours each session.*

I had a control pause of 10 seconds on the 5th, 15 seconds on the 12th. I am now at 32 seconds.

I have been attending Professor [surname] for 30 years. I go to see him twice a year at his rooms in the Elm Park Hospital. I told him I was going for this and asked him his advice. He said: 'Marie, try anything that will help.' I go back to see him in September. He will see a great difference in me. I have a quality of life I have not had for 40 years.

I have been in hospital for an eye operation. The doctors there said my chest was very clear, no cough or mucus. I spend at least four weeks every year in Elm Park so they are used to my condition. I did my exercises while I was in, three times a day. I went on holidays to the Canaries for the month of May, my first holiday in years. I went with my wheelchair. It stayed in my apartment till we were coming home. I did my exercises three times per day and walked two miles every day, taking a rest about six times.

This method has turned my life around. I use a treadmill for two minutes about six times a day.

I am certain it would help hundreds of people.

Yours sincerely,

Marie [Surname]

What about conventional medicine?

Asthma is now the single most common ailment in the Western world and conventional medicine cannot identify why. In fact, the list of things that conventional medicine has yet to discover about asthma is quite an extensive one, including:

+ What causes asthma.
+ Why various triggers start an attack.
+ What causes inflammation, and why it gets worse.
+ Exactly how steroids work.[1]
+ Why swimming can be beneficial.
+ Why some children grow out of asthma and others don't.
+ Why asthma returns in later life, usually as late onset.

Many of those attending our clinics tell me that they feel greatly let down by the medical community; that was how I felt myself. For a major part of their lives, these people have had to put up with a debilitating condition which has frequently diminished their quality of life. Then they come across this method, or they are told about it by someone who is rarely their doctor. They start paying attention to their breathing and doing the breathing exercises, and they find that they experience a dramatic reduction in their asthma problems. They persist with the various disciplines that Asthma Care requires – breathing exercises, physical exercise, sensible diet – and the improvement continues. Then they wonder why they were not taught this therapy earlier, or at least taught the importance of paying attention to their breathing.

They don't understand why this approach is never mentioned by their doctor. It does after all, adopt a complementary medicine approach and people are always advised to consult their doctors before considering changing their medication levels.

Breath retraining is natural, safe and based on medical physiology, so it makes sense. What could be more natural than calm, silent, regular nasal breathing – rather than the irregular, erratic and sometimes noisy mouth breathing that is typical of many asthmatics, even though they may not be aware of it?

To date, this therapy has received positive feedback from thousands of people worldwide who have experienced lasting relief from their asthma symptoms. It is the much maligned media who have been instrumental in creating greater awareness of Buteyko for asthmatics in Australia, New Zealand, Britain and Ireland, in particular by featuring people who have successfully applied this therapy.

But many people remain sceptical, and understandably so when there is so little interest in, never mind support for Buteyko from the medical profession. Why is this? And more to the point in this era of financial constraints and health service cutbacks, why is there a total lack of interest from the Department of Health? The annual cost of asthma to both the patient and State is estimated to be €463 million and this figure increases every year. Furthermore, the average estimated cost to each patient is €1,711, although this figure almost doubles for more severely affected patients.[2]

While all this money is being spent every year by individual patients and the State, a tried and tested method of helping people to solve their own asthma problems naturally, and at no cost to the taxpayer, is ignored.

Why correct your breathing?

As previously stated, my main purpose in writing this book is to spread the word about the benefits of breathing a correct volume of air. It has been of enormous benefit to me and naturally I would like other asthma sufferers to enjoy the same benefits.

If more people hear about the method and decide to take advice on it, then it's likely that my practice will prosper. Therefore, it could be argued easily that I have a vested interest in converting more people with asthma into devotees. There's no point in being disingenuous; it may be the case that I do have a vested interest, but I also have a genuine desire to inform more people about correct breathing, and my motivation is not primarily commercial.

I already know from personal experience what it is like to suffer from chronic asthma. I already know what it's like to take control of it too and, if Asthma Care is about anything, it is about **enabling people to take control of their own asthma problem**. If a patient successfully follows the advice he or she gets then that patient will not need to see me again. There is no magic bottle, no elixir, and no expensive therapy. Asthma sufferers are given practical advice and information, and that's it.

But what happens in the case of your normal medication? I recall being told by my doctor casually, as he wrote a prescription for me, that 'you'll be taking these for the rest of your life'.

Read the leaflet that comes with your asthma medication: 'Do not stop taking this medication without consulting your doctor.' A dependency has been created. The experience of most asthma sufferers is that the medication gets stronger and stronger over the years, but so does the asthma problem. This is a classic addiction cycle.

When they're asked about the Buteyko Clinic Method, respiratory consultants will state that there has been very little research on the method, and what does exist now is only a small number of trials and pilot studies. Naturally, consultants therefore tend to shy away from advising patients to try the method.

Why the lack of research?

Good question. On July 23rd, 2003 *Sky News* reported 'Glaxo Boosts Profits' with the following figures: 'The profits of £3.55 billion, equivalent to £242 per second, came despite seeing generic versions of its antibiotic Augmentin hit US sales of the drug by almost £300 million over the six-month period. **But its asthma drug Seretide boosted earnings with sales worth more than £1 billion in the first half [of the year] – an increase of thirty-nine per cent.'** [Author's emphasis.]

One model of this inhaler (Seretide 250mcg) is now widely prescribed in Ireland and costs €120 per monthly unit. One billion pounds is an enormous amount of money, but who is paying over this huge sum to Glaxo? People with asthma; in other words people like you, that's who.

Most medical research is either conducted or funded by the pharmaceutical industry. A successful research programme will result in a product that generates a substantial income stream for the company in question. The pharmaceutical industry, like any other industry, is driven by the need to increase shareholder value; in other words, there is the need to generate more and more profit every year. If research verifies the validity of reversal of hyperventilation, no multi-million product results. In fact the outcome is quite the reverse: a lot of very expensive asthma treatment products become obsolete, income is reduced, and profits take what would probably be a very big hit. No pharmaceutical company is going to go down that road.

The prevailing wisdom is that turkeys won't vote for Christmas. Pharmaceutical companies are even smarter than turkeys.

It is an unfortunate business fact that the pharmaceutical industry has a vested interest in an increasing asthma population, and the resultant increasing demand for increasingly expensive asthma medication. This is true of any medical problem: the bigger the problem the bigger the profit.

Back in the peace and love days of the '60s, Tom Paxton wrote a line in a song: *'Peace hurts business and that ain't right'*. Good health hurts business too and it still ain't right, but it is seen as the natural order of things.

The lack of establishment support for, or even interest in trials was highlighted during the 1998 BBC television programme Q̲ED, which by way of conclusion posed the question: 'Will anyone give this treatment a proper trial?'[3]

The pharmaceutical industry is not a collection of monsters and ogres; it largely consists of men and women, some of them very dedicated scientists with honourable motives, doing the best they can for their employers, just as most of us do every day. They do a very good job in many respects, so much so that the bigger companies in the industry are extremely successful and, as a result, financially very strong. As a consequence of good stewardship resulting in company strength, they have also become very, very powerful. Many, including myself, would argue that pharmaceutical companies have become too powerful.

I hope I have explained why these companies are unlikely to support objective research into the area of hypoventilation (reduced breathing).

And the doctors?

I have a certain amount of sympathy for doctors in all this. Most doctors that I know work long hours dealing with huge numbers of patients, all of whom are concerned about their health, and at least some of whom are very demanding. Most patients want quick and easy solutions.

One result of the long hours is that many doctors have insufficient time to upgrade their own knowledge or research developments. Pharmaceutical companies subject them to a veritable bombardment of information about new and improved drugs. They are told how these drugs have performed in trials and tests, about the research that has gone into them, and they receive free samples of the drugs. There has even been a suggestion that some asthma nurses who provide clinics at doctors' surgeries in Ireland may be the direct employees of drug companies. Doctors prescribe these drugs if they feel they can help their patients. By and large the system seems to work and people's health does improve – even if they frequently find that they depend on a drug to maintain the improvement.

One result of this virtual indoctrination is that, as with most skilfully targeted marketing campaigns, after a while you believe the claims being made in spite of yourself.

Doctors can only rely on the research results they are given or that they read about. In the circumstances perhaps it is understandable that they are wary of suggesting the Buteyko approach to their patients. There is also the problem that many people will not be prepared to accept the discipline that it requires, and should the method prove unsuccessful for this reason they would blame the doctor; Ireland being such a litigious country they may also sue.

However it is my opinion that doctors owe it to their patients at least to enquire into something like the Buteyko Method which has such a well-documented history of success and such a medically valid basis. Where they are confident that a particular patient will undertake the discipline, they should at least tell him or her about it.

The role of Government

In my view, our Government in general and the Department
of Health in particular, are where the real problem lies, and
also the only solution. The pharmaceutical industry isn't
going to change, and doctors still need research data that
they feel they can trust. The old regime in Russia could make
the sort of radical change that was needed because of the
political system, and also because they couldn't afford
the Western approach. Remember that Russia is where the
method has been most widely and most successfully used.

What is needed is **independent, Government-funded
research** into the Buteyko Method. By Government-funded
research, I mean research not funded even indirectly by
pharmaceutical companies, and not influenced in any way by
them either.

There is an enormous potential saving here for the
national finances of hundreds of millions of euro, and that's
your money and mine. There is potentially the same saving
again for asthma sufferers individually. There would be a
further saving for industry in terms of less absenteeism, a
development that would improve the Irish economy generally.

How much would such a research programme cost? I
don't know, but when you look at the potential savings in
terms of money alone, never mind the substantial improvement in people's basic health and quality of life, the case for
research funding seems unanswerable.

I am asking people with asthma to tackle their TD and
ask him or her to take it up with the Minister for Health and,

equally importantly, with the Minister for Finance. Governments understand money much better than they understand health issues.

However, I predict that there will be huge resistance to the idea of allocating scarce resources to the research of hyperventilation. That resistance will come primarily from pharmaceutical companies that have large manufacturing facilities in Ireland. These companies give very good employment to substantial numbers of people and therefore have a lot of influence at Government level. They also have big PR budgets to ensure they get their message across. Multinational companies are powerful, and sometimes ruthless, entities. Asthma medication is a huge money-spinner for them and nobody likes a threat to their income. TDs with pharmaceutical plants in their constituencies will be especially vulnerable to the threat of job losses.

That being said, it's our health and increasingly our children's health we're talking about. Do we really want to condemn our own children to a life of drug dependency? That is what the medication route means. Will we continue to accept the hugely expensive and spectacularly unsuccessful drug-based approach? I hope not, but I fear so.

And yet if the will is there it's amazing what can be achieved.

The role of the individual

Even if we don't persuade those in power to back Government-funded and independent research, what else can be done? To be more specific, what can you do? Yes, I do mean you, the individual asthma sufferer who is reading this book. My suggestion is that when you have finished reading this book, talk to your doctor and give it a go. If you have found this book to be heavy going or if you want more information, I suggest that you contact a Buteyko practitioner and your doctor. Either way give it a try; remember, you've nothing to lose except your asthma problem.

However, you must be prepared to change your ways. There is a certain amount of discipline involved: you will have to do the breathing exercises, take the modest amount of physical exercise that is required, and you may have to change to a more sensible diet.

Believe me, the rewards more than justify the effort. Nothing worthwhile ever comes easy.

Conclusion

By reading this book, you have taken the first step towards changing your asthma condition forever. It will take time so be patient; it will take determination so persevere; it will take observation so be aware.

Remember, it doesn't matter what new therapies, vaccinations, gene discoveries, medications or other treatments are developed. As long as overbreathing is not addressed, a fundamental and crucial part of the management of asthma is ignored. In my opinion it is now time to educate the Western world to the detrimental effects of overbreathing.

Breathing is the only function of critical importance over which we can exercise control. We cannot voluntarily increase oxygen and blood flow to tissues and organs; we cannot voluntarily reduce our blood pressure; we cannot voluntarily order the airways to open, but we can influence all these vital functions by addressing an incorrect breathing pattern.

The general belief is that big breathing is a result of asthma. In this book, I have demonstrated that the opposite is the case. Big breathing causes loss of carbon dioxide. The body's main defence mechanism against this is to narrow the airways to prevent further loss of carbon dioxide. We struggle to draw in even more air. The cycle begins.

In this book, I have tried to encourage you to become more aware of your breathing. I also have drawn your attention to the well-established relationship between incorrect breathing and your asthma. Normally we do not have to remember to breathe in and out; it happens naturally. So it is probable that this will be the first time in your life that you will be so observant of and aware of your breathing. At the same time however, it is possible to exercise a measure of control over our breathing: we can change the volume, and we can also influence the rate, within certain parameters.

I have included here many exercises that can be self taught. However some of the exercises are a simplified version of those that would be taught at Asthma Care Clinics workshops. This is because it is important that they are done properly, and without feedback it can be difficult to know whether or not the technique is correct. In other cases exercises have only been included in part because it is difficult to communicate them solely by the written word, and misinterpretation may only exacerbate your symptoms.

Ideally, the best way to guarantee a permanent improvement in your asthma is to avail of the services of a qualified and experienced practitioner, preferably one who has an indepth knowledge and understanding of asthma. Your practitioner will give you the tools, the motivation and the follow-up support necessary to make this life-long change. In addition, a well qualified practitioner will tailor exercises to your condition, ensure that you are able to practice them correctly and get you to your destination via the shortest route possible. Having said that, when applied correctly much of the information contained throughout this book will bring about a noticeable improvement in your condition.

If you are a parent reading this book and you have an asthmatic child in the family, you can start applying the basics of this therapy immediately. I truly believe that there is no greater gift that you can give an asthmatic child. Encourage nasal breathing, do not over-clothe them, don't let them overeat – indeed, try to encourage them to eat sensibly – and instil the importance of breathing 'as if they are not breathing'. All this is easier said than done, I know, but if you can convey the facts to children simply and honestly, they should appreciate that this approach will help their asthma problem.

If you complete the exercises in this book and there is no improvement, or even a deterioration, in your asthma then you may not be doing the exercises correctly. In this situation it would be better to stop doing the exercises and contact a Buteyko practitioner. The Buteyko Method is not about taking risks with your asthma, so don't take any risks and don't cause yourself distress. Always take your preventer medication as prescribed and carry a reliever inhaler in case you need it. All too often, asthmatics deny the true extent of their condition and as a result leave themselves prone to a very serious attack. Each year, many hundreds and thousands of people around the world die unnecessarily from asthma attacks.

You now have the tools to take control of your asthma naturally, safely and effectively. Start applying them. Do what you can to help your condition. It is your life and your health, and the power rests within you.

Now I have a final request to make. When your asthma symptoms decrease and you are finally able to take control of your condition by reversing your hyperventilation, I ask you to tell your doctor, your local branch of the Asthma Society, the Minister for Health and anyone else who comes to mind about the improvement in your asthma and how it was achieved. If enough people do this, it may encourage more medical professionals to begin taking an interest in what is being achieved by breath retraining. I feel that we have an obligation to our children to minimise the amount of unnecessary medication we allow them to be given. Adult asthma sufferers deserve no less too, but adults are in a position to make their own choices.

I want to close by wishing you every success in using this approach to help you and your children with breath retraining, and I hope that this book will help as many people as possible to gain control of their asthma with minimal or no medication.

Naturally.

'To tell the truth is not only a responsibility to yourself and others. It is an honour, a duty and your legacy to the generations to come. It is part of their rightful inheritance.'

– Unknown

hyperventilation

This section is a simple explanation of the theory of over-breathing and the role of carbon dioxide in the body. There's no medical jargon here, but the information may seem a little complex simply because it's not everyday reading material. My advice is to read through this section slowly and return to it occasionally.

You don't need to know this information off by heart, but it is important to at least have a basic understanding of the theory. In my experience, people who apply breathing exercises without having a good understanding of the concept of overbreathing and the role of carbon dioxide do not receive the full benefits.

Buteyko Clinic Method

Over four decades, Russian scientist Professor Konstantin Buteyko completed pioneering work on illnesses that develop as a result of breathing more air than the body needs. His life's vocation provided humanity with what is arguably the greatest discovery to date in the field of medicine.

As a medical student, he discovered from his observations of hundreds of patients that their breathing was closely related to the extent of their illnesses. The greater the volume of air inhaled by a patient, the worse the sickness, he noted. This newly-discovered relationship between breathing and health was so precise that he was even able to predict accurately the exact time sick patients would pass away.

As a result of his research, Buteyko went on to devise a breathing programme for his patients, based on reducing the amount of air that passed through their lungs. When each patient applied reduced breathing, all physiological functions including pulse, volume of breathing per minute and blood pressure were monitored. As time went on, the results helped Buteyko to refine and improve his method.

His theory is based on breathing, the life force of any organisim. We humans can live without water and food for many days and weeks but we cannot live without air for more than a few minutes. One wonders then why something so vital to life receives so little attention.

It can often take many years before a medical discovery is acknowledged and incorporated into everyday practice. This was the case with Buteyko's theory, but his experience is reflected through medical and world history. For example, Professor Lister discovered that many illnesses such as sepsis could be passed from doctor to patient by the contaminated hands of the doctor. Lister tested his hypothesis by disinfecting his hands prior to each operation and this resulted in a decrease in the death rate of his patients. It took many years for this discovery to be accepted by the medical community who only did so when patients' relatives started demanding that doctors disinfect their hands before operating.

Although research conducted in Russia in 1962 proved unequivocally the soundness of Buteyko's Method, it was not until 1983 that the Committee on Inventions and Discoveries formally acknowledged his work. This recognition, which begs the question of how many more people would have benefited from the discovery if it was acknowledged earlier, was backdated to January 29th, 1962.

Buteyko's discovery on October 7th, 1952 has improved the health and saved the lives of many thousands of people. Now that his discovery is becoming better known in the Western world, it will save the lives of many more.

Breathing volume

Clinically, overbreathing is known as hyperventilation which means breathing more air than the body needs. If this is happening on a day-to-day basis, it is called chronic hyperventilation. 'Hyper' means over and 'ventilation' means breathing.

The standard volume of normal breathing for a healthy person is three to five litres of air per minute. During an asthma or panic attack, this breathing level can increase to more than twenty litres per minute, a level which is detrimental to health and unsustainable for a lengthy period. Less obvious and more prevalent is habitually breathing a volume of between five and twenty litres per minute. Based on genetic factors, according to Professor Buteyko, this results in an individual developing illness.

Severe overbreathing can be fatal if it is sustained over a short period of time, so it is plausible to accept that there will be negative health effects caused by less severe but still excessive breathing over a long period of time. Long-term overbreathing leads to the build-up of organ damage, resulting in the development of illnesses specific to the hereditary traits of each person. Professor Buteyko's Method restores correct carbon dioxide levels and therefore leads to an overall improvement in general health.

In Russia, this therapy is practised by an estimated two hundred qualified medical doctors in the treatment of a hundred varied illnesses including hypertension, tinnitus, diabetes, and hypo/ hyperthyroidism. The results of treating asthma with the Buteyko Method are swift, so it is used in the West mainly in the treatment of this condition.

Volume of breathing of a person with asthma

Scientific research conducted by Professor Buteyko over three decades and scientific trials at the Mater Hospital in Brisbane in 1995 demonstrated **that people with asthma breathe a volume of ten to twenty litres per minute between attacks and over twenty litres during an attack**. For example, the average volume of air measured during the Mater Hospital Buteyko Trials was 14.1 litres per minute, although other researchers showed a volume of 15 litres (*Johnson et al 1995*) and 12 litres (*McFadden & Lyons 1968*).

Often, overbreathing is not obvious or noticeable and therefore was called 'hidden hyperventilation' by Professor

Buteyko. Other researchers, such as Robert Fried in his book *Hyperventilation Syndrome*, have agreed with this description. In addition, hidden ventilation has been observed at my own Asthma Care Clinic; many people show no outward signs of hyperventilating, yet their asthma as indicated by history and drug regime may be quite serious. These same people benefit significantly from exercises aimed at reversing hyperventilation.

Earlier in this book, we learned a simple way of measuring the extent of our overbreathing by performing a simple test developed by Professor Buteyko called the control pause. As overbreathing is related to the extent of our illness, we can determine the state of our asthma by our control pause. An improvement of the control pause coincides with improvement in our condition.

Carbon dioxide

Ever since Lavoisier proved in the eighteenth century that oxygen was essential to life, carbon dioxide – which is an end product of our metabolism – became known as a waste gas. Lavoisier compared bodily functions to the process of fire; both fire and the human body absorb oxygen and produce carbon dioxide and heat.

The sustenance of life requires oxygen and carbon dioxide. Just as excess oxygen results in damage to the lungs when the toxicity level is higher than antioxidants can counteract, too little carbon dioxide impairs the correct functioning of all organs.

The key to Buteyko theory is that carbon dioxide is not just a waste gas; it is essential for all metabolic functions. Dr Yandell Henderson put it well when he wrote: *'carbon dioxide is the chief hormone of the entire body, it is the only one that is produced by every tissue and that probably acts on every organ,'* in the Cyclopedia of Medicine published in 1940.

Evolution of the lungs and atmospheric changes of carbon dioxide

An estimated five hundred million years ago, when the first prototype of human lungs evolved, the level of carbon dioxide in the atmosphere was approximately twenty per cent. This high concentration was due to excessive volcanic activity which produced CO_2 in abundance, and a scarcity of plant life meant that such a large quantity was not absorbed and recycled.

Over millions of years, the amount of plant life on earth increased and carbon dioxide levels continued to decline to the present day rate of just .035 per cent. Our lungs adapted to less carbon dioxide by creating air sacs to retain the higher amount of five to six-and-a-half per cent necessary for human life. The womb is a perfect environment for the survival of human life, and it contains a carbon dioxide concentration of between seven and eight per cent.

How does overbreathing affect carbon dioxide?

If you breathe in a large volume of air then you will breathe out a large volume. Humans don't inhale air to store it in any form in the body, so therefore the volume exhaled has to be the same as the volume inhaled.

Exhaling a large volume of air results in too much carbon dioxide being carried from the alveoli within our lungs and into the atmosphere. To understand this, imagine a plastic straw. Place tiny droplets of water along the inside of the imaginary straw. You already know that if you breathe out very gently through the straw, you will not blow out these little droplets of water. However, if you breathe out very quickly, the quantity of air you exhale will carry the droplets of water out with it. This is similar to what happens in our lungs; the more air we inhale causes more air to be exhaled, and this greater quantity of exhaled air results in too much carbon dioxide being carried out of the body.

Medical science has long recognised that the required amount of carbon dioxide in the little air sacs of the lungs, the alveoli, for a healthy person is between five and six-and-a-half per cent. This is well illustrated in any university medical textbook. However, constant overbreathing leads to a loss of carbon dioxide and the concentration may drop as low as three-and-a-half per cent. Butekyo found that a level of below three per cent led to death.

Carbon dioxide fixed at incorrect level

Under normal conditions, the respiratory centre located in our brain – called central chemoreceptors – instructs us to breathe based not on the level of oxygen, but on the level of carbon dioxide. Oxygen only becomes the main stimulant driving respiration when its concentration becomes very low, as in the event of asphyxiation.

The way our respiratory centre works is easily explained by comparing it to a household heating thermostat. We set the thermostat at the desired temperature and when the temperature goes below this level, the heating system switches on. When the room warms up to the desired level, the thermostat sends an instruction to switch the heating off again.

Our respiratory centre is the regulator or thermostat for our carbon dioxide. When the level of carbon dioxide goes below the amount set by the respiratory centre, a message is sent to decrease breathing to restore the level of the gas in the body. Decreasing breathing results in an accumulation of carbon dioxide, thus restoring it to set levels. Likewise, when the level of carbon dioxide is higher than the amount set by the respiratory centre, a message is sent to increase breathing. This increased breathing blows off the additional carbon dioxide and brings it back to the level set by the regulator.

However, breathing more than your body needs over a period of hours, weeks, months, or years will result in the day-to-day levels of carbon dioxide remaining low. Our respiratory centre becomes accustomed to or fixed at this lower level of carbon dioxide and determines it to be 'correct'. Our respiratory centre will therefore instruct us to overbreathe to maintain this low level of carbon dioxide, even though the rest of the body's organs and tissues are suffering.

Reversing hyperventilation is achieved both by observing our breathing and by practising exercises to recondition the body to accept a higher but more correct level of carbon dioxide. Essentially hyperventilation is a bad habit which we aim to change.

If a patient can't understand that their asthma is being caused by overbreathing, a hyperventilation provocation test can prove useful. The patient is instructed to take many big breaths, as if they had just finished a race. Generally within two minutes, the patient will start to feel the onset of symptoms such as chest tightness, blocked nose, wheezing and coughing. When the symptoms begin, the patient is instructed to reduce breathing and the symptoms reverse. In practice, about seventy per cent of patients will experience symptoms from deliberate hyperventilation within two minutes. Naturally, this technique is used only as a last resort to prove to the patient that symptoms are a direct result of overbreathing; the patient is always instructed to stop hyperventilating well in advance of an attack. It is not advisable to practise this test without medical supervision.

Why is carbon dioxide so important?

Carbon dioxide is essential to human life. Loss of it due to overbreathing is, according to Professor Buteyko, the primary cause of asthma. For people who are predisposed to developing asthma, maintaining the correct level of carbon dioxide is very important for the following reasons:

✦ Transportation of oxygen

Oxygen is relatively insoluble in blood, so ninety-eight per cent of the gas is carried by haemoglobin molecule. The release of oxygen from haemoglobin is dependent on the quantity of carbon dioxide in our alveoli/arterial blood. If the level of carbon dioxide is not at the required level of five to six-and-a-half per cent, oxygen has a stronger 'bond' to haemoglobin and so is not released to tissues and organs.

What this means is that oxygen is being carried with the blood on a round trip around your body, without reaching its proper destinations such as the cells, tissues and organs. A vicious circle ensues because low oxygen levels will stimulate the respiratory centre, leading to a further increase in breathing and loss of carbon dioxide ... such as during an asthma attack.

This bond was named after the two physicians who discovered it and is now known as the Bohr Werigo Effect. It is important to know that blood is ninety-eight per cent saturated with oxygen at a breathing volume of three to five litres of air per minute.

✦ Dilation of blood vessels

Carbon dioxide dilates the smooth muscle around airways, arteries and capillaries. Reduced carbon dioxide causes smooth muscle to constrict, so people genetically predisposed to develop asthma have greater narrowing of the airways. Reduced carbon dioxide also results in arteries and capillaries constricting. When arteries and capillaries narrow, the heart must work harder to distribute blood throughout the body, resulting in increased heart beat and for some people higher blood pressure. Following an increase in carbon dioxide, there is greater oxygenation of body cells and tissues due to the dilation of blood vessels. Instant feedback comes in the form of reduced symptoms and increased body warmth due to improved blood circulation.

+ **Maintaining PH balance**

It is very important that the human body stays within normal acid/alkali (PH) balance. Acid PH is measured from one to seven, with one being much more acidic. Alkaline PH is measured from seven to fourteen, with the most alkaline being fourteen. Neutral PH is seven.

The human body requires a slightly alkaline PH of 7.365 on this scale of one to fourteen, and even small shifts in the body's PH balance can be catastrophic. According to the eighth edition of Guyton's Medical Physiology textbook: *'The lower limit at which a person can live more than a few hours is about 6.8 and the upper limit approximately 8.0'.*

When carbon dioxide leaves the lungs, the body becomes more alkaline resulting in reduced metabolic functioning and poorer immunity. Professor Buteyko believes that inflammation and allergic hyper-responsiveness is caused by an immune system which does not function correctly due to low carbon dioxide.

Pollen, dust mites, allergens, stress, and other asthma triggers are not the cause of asthma. They trigger an attack when the immune system is already hypersensitive. People with a poor immune system are also more susceptible to developing colds and flu. When the immune system is strengthened, triggers no longer cause an attack and there is a significant reduction in the incidences of colds and flu.

✦ Maintaining nature's steroid

Cortisol is the body's natural steroid. Hyperventilation causes an inadequate production of cortisol. When the body is not producing enough to meet its own needs, then it must be supplemented with synthetic drugs such as Becotide or Flixotide. When hyperventilation is reversed, adrenal functioning improves and leads to less need for steroidal medication. This has been proven in the Mater Hospital trials held in Brisbane in 1995, which concluded that there was 50 per cent less need for steroid medication when hyperventilation was reduced. Furthermore, those who reduced their breathing volume the most were able to reduce their steroid intake the most.

✦ Controlling mucus production

Mucus forms an important part of the body's defence system by trapping foreign particles and invaders, and deactivating them before they reach the lungs. Mucus is constantly brushed up to the throat by tiny hair-like structures called cilia, thus removing potential threats. When carbon dioxide is low, the body produces more mucus. While mucus plays an essential role in the airways, excessive mucus narrows the airways and results in greater breathing difficulty.

A combination of all these factors leads to the classical asthma symptoms of chest tightness, coughing, excess mucus production, wheezing, shortness of breath, nasal problems, sleep problems and lethargy. Buteyko cites asthma as the body's defence to stop and reduce the amount of carbon dioxide being lost. When carbon dioxide increases to normal, the defence mechanism is no longer needed, and the result is no asthma symptoms.

Therefore correct carbon dioxide levels result in:

+ Greater oxygenation of tissues and organs due to Bohr Werigo effect.
+ More open airways thus allowing unrestricted breathing.
+ Better immune system functioning. For example, the immune system is strong enough to withstand colds and infections but not hypersensitive enough to perceive harmless particles such as dust mites, pollens and other triggers as threats.
+ More adequate production of cortisol, the natural steroid necessary to control inflammation.
+ Less mucus production resulting in less restricted airways.

Why do I have asthma?

Professor Buteyko believes that genetic predisposition determines which illnesses people develop from overbreathing. The response of each individual to hyperventilation depends on inherited factors.

Various estimates exist regarding the extent of over-breathing among the general population, ranging from thirty per cent, according to Claude Lum, to Sasha Stalmatski's ninety per cent. In Russia, the Buteyko Method is used in the treatment of up to one hundred diseases including hypertension, asthma, bronchitis, emphysema, diabetes and Raynaud's Syndrome.

Carbon dioxide is so important for normal bodily functioning that it is logical to assume the body must have some way to prevent losing it. Narrowing of the airways is a natural defence mechanism present in people with asthma to help maintain carbon dioxide, and it's activated when the level of the gas falls too low. Inflammation, by constriction of smooth muscle and by increased mucus secretion, causes narrowing of the airways.

This might seem a peculiar statement, but people with asthma are better off than the rest of the overbreathers because they are equipped with an instant mechanism to prevent the loss of carbon dioxide. People who do not have this mechanism suffer from many of the incurable diseases of civilisation.

At this point, it is worth noting that before the 1900s people who had asthma often lived longer than the rest of the population, and that death from asthma was unknown. As Professor Buteyko put it: *'Having asthma generally meant having a long life free from many diseases, but nobody could explain why asthma prevented other diseases or why asthmatics lived longer than other people.'* At the end of the nineteenth century, Professor of Medicine at Oxford University Sir William Osler, in his textbook *The*

Principles and Practice of Medicine noted: 'We have no knowledge of the morbid anatomy of true asthma. Death during the attack is unknown.'

Overbreathing resulting from modern living is the cause of breathing-related diseases. Hyperventilation is not a result of asthma; it is the cause of asthma. Reducing hyperventilation leads to a corresponding reversal of asthma. This was confirmed during Professor Buteyko's forty years of research and during independent trials at the Mater Hospital in Brisbane, Australia.

Buteyko believes that people genetically predisposed to asthma will develop asthma only if they are overbreathing. Years ago, people ate less processed food and more vegetation; they physically worked and played more; they were under less stress, and less chemicals and pesticides were used in food production. As a result, people produced more carbon dioxide from physical activity and retained it due to a more correct volume of breathing.

Symptoms of overbreathing or hyperventilation

Hyperventilation contributes to many conditions, but because it receives very little attention in the diagnoses of illnesses, many patients suffering from various physical symptoms sometimes spend years going from doctor to doctor looking for the cause. This group of patients are often labelled as 'psychosomatic' and there is a belief that the condition is 'all in the head'.

Physician Claude Lum noted that hyperventilation '*presents a collection of bizarre and often apparently unrelated symptoms, which may affect any part of the body, any organ and any system*'.

Some of the symptoms of hyperventilation affect:

+ **The respiratory system** in the form of wheezing, breathlessness, coughing, chest tightness, frequent yawning and snoring.

+ **The nervous system** in the form of a light-headed feeling, poor concentration, numbness, sweating, dizziness, vertigo, tingling of hands and feet, faintness, trembling and headache.

+ **The heart**, typically a racing heartbeat, pain in the chest region, and a skipping or irregular heartbeat.

+ **The mind**, including some degrees of anxiety, tension, depression, apprehension and stress.

+ **Other general symptoms** include mouth dryness, fatigue, bad dreams, nightmares, dry itchy skin, sweaty palms, increased urination such as bed wetting or regular visits to the bathroom during the night, diarrhoea, constipation, general weakness and chronic exhaustion.

Why do we overbreathe?

Earlier on I explained that when we overbreathe on a permanent basis, the respiratory centre in our brain is trained to accept a lower level of carbon dioxide. This level is determined to be correct even though it is less than the body requires for good health. The respiratory centre is like a loyal servant who adapts to changing circumstances and situations for its master.

There are many reasons why we overbreathe but not all of them may apply to each individual. The following ten factors are more prevalent in countries of increasing modernisation and affluence, and this helps explain why asthma and other diseases of civilisation are so prevalent in the same countries.

1. Breathing exercises during pregnancy

Women during pregnancy are taught deep breathing exercises throughout countries in the Western world. This excessive breathing reduces the woman's level of carbon dioxide. As the embryo receives all its nutrients from the mother, her embryo will also obtain less carbon dioxide. Professor Buteyko claimed that the reason many babies suffer from various conditions such as asthma and eczema is because of their mothers' hyperventilation during pregnancy. After birth, the baby may be over-clothed and raised on formula foods. These factors also contribute to sustaining the loss of carbon dioxide that began during pregnancy.

2. Diet

Over-eating increases breathing because the body requires more energy to digest and process food. Instead of listening to the body and eating when hungry, as we have done for thousands of years, society now dictates at what time we should eat. In addition, we condition ourselves to eat more food than is necessary. How many times have you continued

to eat all the food on your plate, or all the courses on offer,
even though you didn't feel hungry?

We have lost the art of listening to the body about what
it needs. People in ancient times only ate when they were
hungry. The primary reason for this was that hunting and
gathering food required effort, and that more energy had to
be spent to gather a larger quantity of food. Our ancestors
didn't have the luxury of accessible modern-day convenience
stores, supermarkets and fast-food outlets to obtain something to eat whenever they desired, so they ate less and
better food.

Often, we eat too quickly due to a hectic lifestyle. As
a result, we do not recognise when we have over-eaten
because it takes time for the body to send us the signals to
stop.

Protein, especially animal protein, and processed foods
contribute to overbreathing. Professor Buteyko believes that
food is the single biggest contributor to overbreathing. A
supplementary factor is the use of chemicals and pesticides
in growing all foodstuffs. The body has to work harder
to remove the increased amount of toxins in food. This
increases breathing.

3. Misconception of deep breathing

The traditional view in the Western world is that deep
breathing is conducive to fitness and maintaining good
health. A 'deep breath' is misinterpreted as a 'big breath'. This
fixed belief prevails among sports coaches, schools, hospitals,
asthma clinics, radio, TV, magazines and even Western yoga.
The most common instruction to those taking exercise or

experiencing stress is to 'take a deep breath'. By exercising in the gym or taking a walk along the beach, you can see how many people believe in the benefits of big breathing. At my clinic, I ask each person if he feels that deep breathing is good for him. About seventy per cent of people feel it is and the remainder don't know because they are unconscious of their breathing.

In the Eastern world, reduced breathing and breath control is very much enshrined in culture and philosophy. Its therapeutic value has been recognised for centuries.

4. Stress

Interpreting outside events, often those over which we can have no control, results in stress. Stress can be positive in the form of laughter, for example, or negative in the form of anxiety. Stress activates the sympathetic nervous response known as 'fight or flight'. Throughout evolution, people were often faced with life-threatening situations so human physiology changed in response to these situations in order to ensure survival of the species. During stress, blood is diverted from internal organs to skeletal muscles and respiration increases to prepare the body for increased physical activity. Evolutionary people were therefore ready to fight or take flight, depending on the dangers facing them.

However, our evolution has not kept pace with changes in modern life and our bodies often perform poorly to stress arising from marital problems, financial pressure or everyday situations such as traffic jams or late buses. Breathing is increased by stress, and in turn breathing leads to excitability of many brain areas, resulting in states of anxiety, panic and many psychological problems. At this point, one factor will feed off the other thus maintaining a constant state of arousal.

5. Temperature

Living in a hot and stuffy environment causes overbreathing. While body temperature is primarily controlled by skin pores and sweat glands, wearing too much clothing causes us to revert to primitive mouth panting as a way of regulating temperature.

A child's metabolism is two to three times faster than an adult's and therefore generates more energy. Children have a natural instinct to wear less clothing than adults, and this results in greater freedom and liveliness. We adults, however, dress children according to the temperature we feel ourselves and fail to take into account how warm the children feel, so an individual child who is wearing too many clothes will overbreathe.

Thanks to central heating and PVC windows and doors, our homes are better insulated and are becoming progressively warmer. Years ago houses were less well insulated and cooler, and a draught often brought fresh air through gaps under doors or between window frames. Research has demonstrated that mild or cool environments assist reduced breathing.

6. Lack of physical exercise

Exercise enables the body to accumulate large amounts of carbon dioxide produced by metabolic activity; lack of physical motion means less activity and less carbon dioxide.

For most people now, work means more mental effort and less physical activity. Even most of our forms of entertainment take place indoors, such as cinemas, theatres, computer games and satellite television. Out of an average twenty-four hour day, eight are spent sleeping, fourteen sitting and just two hours standing or walking. Compare this to the average day of our ancestors who spent all their waking hours completing tasks that demanded physical activity.

7. Over-sleeping

Professor Buteyko's research shows that lying down horizontally for a long period of time causes severe overbreathing. Most asthma attacks occur between the hours of 3.00 and 5.00 a.m. when the body's level of carbon dioxide passes below its lower threshold due to excessive breathing during sleep. Professor Buteyko emphasised that the position which causes the most overbreathing is sleeping while lying on one's back. Incidentally, this can be observed among many people who stop snoring when they are turned over onto their side.

8. Pollution

When air is either insufficient or polluted, our bodies sense we are not getting enough air so we breathe more to compensate. Many people with asthma can testify to increased symptoms following time spent in a stuffy or smoky atmosphere.

Pollution itself is not to blame for the rising tide of asthma in developed countries, despite numerous studies and claims to that effect. If this was so, then why would the rate of asthma continue to be so much less in heavily polluted Asian cities such as Bangkok? Another example is the former East Germany where pollution levels were higher but the asthma rate lower than in West Germany. An additional pointer is that some countries have very low pollution levels but high asthma rates; the relatively unpolluted New Zealand has the third highest incidence of asthma in the world.

9. Bronchodilators

Professor Buteyko's belief is that using bronchodilator drugs to relieve asthma symptoms causes hyperventilation. Bronchodilators relax smooth muscle and force open the airways, increasing the volume of air that can be inhaled with each breath. Steroids are preferable as a treatment because Professor Buteyko discovered that they reduce breathing. It is worth noting that increasing use of bronchodilating drugs during the 1980s corresponded with a significant increase in the asthma death rate.

10. Asthma symptoms

The breathing rate and volume during an asthma attack is invariably greater than under normal conditions when no symptoms are present. When an attack occurs over a prolonged period (24 hours), the respiratory centre adjusts to a greater breathing volume and this is maintained even when the attack has passed. A vicious circle ensues as asthma symptoms encourage a greater breathing volume, and this greater breathing volume results in more asthma symptoms.

Professor Buteyko encapsulates his beliefs as follows: *'One needs to eat less, breathe less, sleep less and physically work harder to the sweat of one's brow because this is good. This is a fundamental change, this is true restructuring. This is what we need to do these days.'*

Future treatment of asthma?

It is quite obvious that our current management of asthma is not working. More and more children are developing asthma and no-one in the medical community seems to know why.

More than ever in our history, children are dependent on powerful drugs which they may have to take for the rest of their lives. Professor Buteyko's hyperventilation theory explains exactly what is happening and why the incidence of asthma is greater in developed countries. Scientific research weighs in behind the effects of hyperventilation.

Our genes have not changed in one hundred years. Our lifestyle unfortunately has, and this has increased our breathing to the detriment of our general health.

A step in the right direction would be government funding of research into non-drug methods of treating asthma, such as the Buteyko Clinic Method. Only then will people with asthma be offered a suitable and sustainable non-medication lifeline. To date, most research has been funded by multinational drug empires who have a vested interest, resulting in the neglect of safe, natural non-drug methods. This is a sad state of affairs for all people with asthma.

hyperventilation and asthma

At this point, it's reasonable to ask if there is any evidence available from Western medical experts that helps to clarify the link between hyperventilation and asthma.

A number of scientific and medical papers have been written that prove hyperventilation plays a predominant role in the onset of asthma symptoms. Some experts have argued that asthma symptoms arise because of a loss of carbon dioxide while others cite additional effects of hyperventilation such as water and/or heat loss from the airways. More significant is the existence of a number of studies and papers in the Western world that support the premise of Buteyko's theory.

In an article entitled *Hyperventilation Syndrome and Asthma*, Demeter notes: 'Hyperventilation whether spontaneous or exercise induced, is known to cause asthma.'[1] His study shows that a large number of patients with hyperventilation syndrome also had asthma, and that treatment by bronchodilating drugs and explanation proved to be highly effective in reducing symptoms. The paper lists a number of symptoms of hyperventilation, including chest tightness, dyspnea (difficult breathing), palpitations, dizziness and others with which most asthmatics will be familiar.

Furthermore, Demeter states that these symptoms are the result of hyperventilation rather than its cause.

Demeter possibly offers an explanation as to why hyperventilation syndrome receives very little attention in the treatment of asthma. Firstly, he explains that it is very difficult to make a diagnosis of hyperventilation in laboratory tests and secondly 'no mention is made of any link' between hyperventilation syndrome and asthma.

For a paper by Elshout *et al* which was published in the highly respected medical journal *Thorax*, a study was done to determine what happens to airway resistance when there is an increase of carbon dioxide (hypercapnia) or a decrease (hypocapnia).[2] Altogether, 15 healthy people and 30 with asthma were involved. It was found that an increase of carbon dioxide determined by measuring end tidal CO_2 resulted in a 'significant fall' in airway resistance in both normal and asthmatic subjects. This simply means that an increase of carbon dioxide caused the airways to become less restricted, resulting in a reduction of asthma symptoms.

On the other hand, a carbon dioxide decline did have a negative effect on the airways of asthmatic subjects, but led to no change in the healthy persons. The conclusion drawn was that 'hypocapnia may contribute to airway obstruction in asthmatic patients, even when water and heat loss is prevented.'

So while a loss of carbon dioxide has no affect on individuals without asthma, it does cause airway obstruction leading to asthma symptoms among those with asthma.

In another paper, entitled *The mechanism of bronchoconstriction due to hypocapnia in man*, Sterling writes that 'hypocapnia (loss of carbon dioxide) due to voluntary hyperventilation in man causes increased resistance to airflow'. Furthermore, when subjects inhaled an air mixture containing five per cent carbon dioxide 'bronchoconstriction was prevented, indicating that it had been due to hypocapnia, not to mechanical factors associated with hyperventilation.'[3]

The following is a quotation from a paper entitled *Demonstration and treatment of hyperventilation causing asthma*: 'Hyperventilation, leading to airways cooling, will cause bronchoconstriction in vulnerable individuals' but, 'because attacks of asthma are accompanied by hyperventilation of physiological origin, the role of hyperventilation in causing asthma attacks may be overlooked'.

In the study, a twenty-year-old man with a lifelong history of asthma was taught breathing exercises over a period of five sessions of thirty minutes each over five months. The patient 'resumed physical activities and became capable of performing levels of exercise never previously achieved'. The article concludes that 'this case demonstrates that training in controlled breathing can help patients who hyperventilate to avoid some attacks of asthma'.[4]

Prolonged hyperventilation

We already know that when hyperventilation occurs over a small period of time, it's not a problem. In this situation, the respiratory centre senses the decrease of carbon dioxide and so automatically reduces or stops the breathing process to enable it to restore to preset levels.[5] In this situation therefore, hyperventilation is only a short-term phenomenon.

However, if overbreathing is prolonged over a long period of time, physiological changes occur in the body resulting in hyperventilation becoming a more permanent state.[5] Demeter also supports this when he states 'prolonged hyperventilation (for more than 24 hours) seems to sensitise the brain, leading to a more prolonged hyperventilation.'[1] Hyperventilation becomes habitual or long term, so even when the primary cause is removed, the behaviour is maintained.

Let's amalgamate this with Buteyko's theory. The lifestyle of modern man increases breathing volume which in turn causes a loss of carbon dioxide, resulting in asthma for persons genetically predisposed. As increased respiratory volume is a common symptom of an attack,[6] asthma plays a role in increasing hyperventilation and therefore symptoms. Simply because an asthma attack can occur over a relatively long period of time, the respiratory centre can become used to accepting a lower level of carbon dioxide. In turn, this leads to increased breathing volume over the long term.[1,5] One feeds the other; hyperventilation leads to an increased breathing volume, and this in turn leads to further hyperventilation.

Water and heat loss

Another area not altogether separate from prolonged hyperventilation is that of exercise-induced asthma [EIA]. Exercise-induced asthma affects up to ninety per cent of asthmatics. While the main theories explaining EIA are water loss or cooling of the airways,[7,8,9] Buteyko and others[2,12] cite loss of carbon dioxide. I have concentrated mainly on the theory of carbon dioxide throughout this book because it has already been well researched by Buteyko and is easily understood. However, lets briefly examine water and heat loss theory.

On commencement of physical exercise, the volume of breathing increases. The airways are therefore required to condition a greater volume of air and this causes the dehydration and cooling effect which plays a primary role in producing asthma symptoms. According to Anderson, the greater the volume of ventilation, the greater the loss of water and cooling of the airways and so the greater the severity of bronchoconstriction.[10]

It is very interesting to note that similar effects to EIA can be reproduced by voluntary hyperventilation. In other words, asthmatic symptoms similar to those caused by exercise can be produced by taking in large volumes of air through the mouth over the course of a few minutes.[11,12,13]

Therefore, it can be accepted without question that the volume of air inhaled and the condition of this air plays a noteworthy role in producing symptoms. It is also logical to state that the airways become dryer and cooler with a greater volume of air passing through. This is not just solely applicable to people undergoing exercise; it also relates to the volume of air inhaled during rest.

Another good question

So how does this relate to Professor Buteyko's work? Well, based on the research detailed already in this appendix, we know that increased ventilation causes bronchoconstriction. We also know that the volume of air typically inhaled by an asthmatic during rest is far greater than the accepted normal level. For example, the reported volume as measured in a number of trials was 15 litres[14], 14.1 litres[15] and 12 litres.[16]

In summary, prolonged hyperventilation causes a resetting of the body's acceptable level of carbon dioxide, allowing the respiratory system to maintain chronic overbreathing. This larger volume of breathing is the primary element in producing asthma symptoms. Therefore, breathing exercises aimed at reversing hyperventilation should have a vital role in reducing asthma symptoms.

Quite simply, the more you reverse your overbreathing, the greater the improvement to your asthma. Your control pause will indicate the extent of the correction of your breathing. At forty seconds, your breathing will be corrected and asthma will not be presenting any symptoms. It is as simple as that.

Difficulty of measuring carbon dioxide levels

The role of carbon dioxide in causing asthma has often been a contentious issue among medical professionals, and it is very difficult to prove. Carbon dioxide can be a difficult gas to measure and some methods involve considerable medical risk such as puncturing an artery. More commonly, carbon dioxide is measured by an instrument called a capnograph. A capnograph measures the amount of carbon dioxide in exhaled air, which is equal to the content within the lungs. However, for the following reasons, the measurement of end tidal carbon dioxide is not as straightforward as it would seem:

+ Once a patient is conscious of having their breathing monitored, their breathing rate and depth will change, giving an untrue measurement. If a mask is placed over the person's face, then the mask will create some resistance, thus reducing the volume of air.

+ The length of each breath plays a crucial role in determining the amount of carbon dioxide in exhaled air. For example, if the patient is instructed to exhale a long breath, breathing will slow down, thus increasing the level of carbon dioxide in the blood. This carbon dioxide will enter the measurement chamber and give a high but false reading of carbon dioxide.

+ If the patient is taking small breaths, then air from 'dead space' – the 150ml part of the airways where no exchange of gas takes place and where there is a very low level of carbon dioxide – enters the chamber along with alveolar air from the lungs. This produces a low but false measurement of carbon dioxide.

Can Buteyko Breathing help explain some old practices?

Apart from the evidence documented above, along with positive verbal feedback from many thousands of people worldwide, there is anecdotal evidence which may prove helpful in demonstrating the link between asthma and over-breathing.

Comedy affects asthma

For example, why would asthma get worse following a long period of time talking; fits of laughter;[17,18] a stressful period; a large meal; a night sleeping with the mouth open; being in a stuffy warm environment, or blowing into a peak flow meter or Spirometry a number of times?

Quite simply, all of these cause overbreathing and over-breathing causes asthma symptoms. All people with asthma will intuitively realise the relationship between these events and their symptoms. For example, if you are in stitches of laughter while watching a comedy or funny film, your laughter will involve large inhalations of air through your mouth in between each laugh. In addition, the increased excitement will in turn increase your breathing. It is not uncommon for asthma symptoms to be worse following attendance at a comedy show.

Swimming

It's accepted that swimming is a very beneficial exercise for people with asthma. It's known that the maximal breathing volume per minute is lower during swimming than during other sports such as running or cycling.[19,20,21]

While the effect of reduced asthma symptoms is primarily believed to be due to the inhalation of warm air,[19,20] the role of carbon dioxide can offer a realistic explanation. For example, if inhaling warm air is beneficial, then remaining in the shower under hot water for an hour each day may help to reduce attacks. A more plausible explanation is that during swimming, reduced breathing results in an increase of carbon dioxide causing bronchodilation.

Unfortunately swimmers are not aware of this link and may spend the rest of their day overbreathing or worse – mouth breathing.

Late onset asthma

Late onset asthma is becoming more common among women and it usually occurs following a stressful period. While a person may be overbreathing for their entire life, the additional increase of breathing due to a stressful event can push their carbon dioxide levels to fall and asthma is activated as a defence mechanism. The respiratory centre becomes set at this lower level of carbon dioxide and so breathing is maintained at a high and unhealthy volume.

Affluence

The incidence of asthma increases relative to modern affluence. This is due to the changes in our lifestyle; it isn't anything to do with our genetic make-up, because this takes thousands and millions of years to evolve. What we call modern civilisation culminates in a greater consumption of processed foods, overeating, overclothing, stress and lack of physical activity. All of these factors contribute to overbreathing and are common in countries with the highest incidence of asthma.

Growing out of it

Why do some children grow out of asthma and others don't? Again, Buteyko Breathing can offer a possible explanation for this. Some children automatically and unconsciously reduce their breathing. Those who don't continue to have asthma into adulthood.

Brown paper bag

Doctors used to recommend breathing into and out of a brown paper bag to stop an asthma attack. While this is not an altogether safe practice, it's based on the concept of restoring the carbon dioxide level to dilate the airways. This is based on the same Buteyko Breathing concept – the restoration of CO_2 levels. Buteyko Breathing, however, relies on natural accumulation of carbon dioxide by reduced breathing and so is therefore safer.

controlled Buteyko trials 1995/2003

A therapy is accepted as having therapeutic value when it is proven and verified by independent trials. This appendix provides a brief summary of trials into Buteyko Breathing in the Western world, which were conducted at the Mater Hospital, Brisbane, Australia in 1995 and Gisborne Hospital, New Zealand in 2003.

Summary of blind randomised trial at the Mater Hospital, Brisbane, 1995

Duration: January to April 1995
Trial sample: 39 people
The purpose of the trial was to evaluate the therapeutic benefits of the Buteyko Breathing Method as a treatment for asthma. The trial was funded by a grant from the Australian Association of Asthma Foundations and conducted by Professor Charles Mitchell.

Following publicity by the Asthma Foundation, one-hundred-and-seventy subjects were interviewed and screened. The forty-two subjects who met the requirements were monitored for a period of four weeks prior to the trial to determine their peak flow readings, medication use and asthma stability. During this period, three subjects were excluded because they did not require sufficient short-acting reliever medication.

Thirty-nine subjects participated in the trial; nineteen were allocated to the Buteyko group and twenty to the control group. Participants were allocated to either group by random selection. There were no significant medication use or airway obstruction differences between either group.

Background

The trial was blind, meaning that none of the participants involved was aware of what therapy he or she was being taught; no mention of Buteyko was made during the training on which the trial results were based.

Buteyko Breathing was taught in accordance with normal Buteyko procedures. The Buteyko practitioner made follow-up calls to each patient as needed, and some participants were given follow-up instruction.

The control group was taught conventional abdominal breathing exercises and relaxation techniques by a physiotherapist. The practitioner in the control group made one call to each participant.

Each participant was instructed to use his or her short-acting reliever medication only as needed. In the event that the requirement for short-acting reliever was reduced to one dose or less per day, participants were instructed to reduce their steroid intake.

All participants completed an individual diary of progress including medication intake and symptoms. Each participant completed quality-of-life questionnaires twice: once when the trial started and again three months later as a comparison measure. The quality-of-life measurement took four indicators into account including mood, breathing, social interaction and concern for others.

Trial results

Exacerbation of symptoms

During the three months of the study, three subjects from each group were admitted to hospital. In addition, six subjects from the Buteyko Method group and seven subjects from the control group received short courses of oral steroids. An approximate number of severe chronic asthmatics were involved in both groups.

Medication usage after three months

Buteyko Group

Average reduction in reliever use:	90%
Average reduction in steroid use:	49%
Daily symptom score:	71% improvement

Control Group

Average reduction in reliever use:	14.78%
Average reduction in steroid use:	0%
Daily symptom score:	14% improvement

Changes in minute volume

Buteyko Group

Average breathing volume per minute at start of trial:	14.1 litres
Average breathing volume after three months:	9.6 litres

Control Group

Average breathing volume per minute at start of trial:	14.2 litres
Average breathing volume after three months:	13.3 litres

[Sources of information in relation to the trials include personal correspondence with the Buteyko practitioner involved, Tess Graham; the *Australia Medical Journal*[1] and the *James Hooper Manual.*[2]]

Conclusions

The Buteyko Breathing group experienced a significant reduction in the need for reliever medication and steroids, along with a greater improvement in quality of life.

The control group showed little change in medication and quality of life despite being taught the conventional breathing exercises that continue to be the mainstay of treatment in hospitals and clinics.

It is interesting to note that half the control group was later taught Buteyko Breathing and the results from this group were consistent with earlier findings, according to Tess Graham, the Buteyko practitioner involved in the trials.

In order to measure only changes to lung function brought about by Buteyko Breathing, preventer medication would be required to remain constant. A reduction of preventer medication generally would lead to a decrease of lung function for any asthmatic. During this trial, the Buteyko group were able to reduce their need for preventer medication and yet there was no deterioration in lung function. In twelve weeks, patients could produce the same lung function scores as before the trial but with less than half the need for medication.

A headline from an article published in *Australian Doctor* read 'Doctors gasp at Buteyko success'. Dr Simon Bowler, a respiratory physician at Mater Hospital in Brisbane was quoted as saying 'we were surpised at the results, as we didn't expect any significant changes.'[3]

Final note

When the trial started, the average volume per minute in the Buteyko group was 14.1 litres and 14.2 litres in the control group. After three months, the average volume per minute was reduced to 9.6 litres in the Buteyko group and 13.3 litres in the control group.

There was a direct correlation between the reduction in use of short-acting reliever and volume per minute of breathing. Those who reduced their breathing volume the most were able to reduce their symptoms – and therefore their medication – the most. In addition, no contraindications or dangers were cited throughout the trials or during the reviews afterwards.

Buteyko's theory is that because hyperventilation causes asthma, a reduction in overbreathing results in a reduction of asthma severity and therefore the need for medication. This was indeed proven by the trials.

Summary of blind randomised controlled trial investigating the efficacy of the Buteyko Method at Gisborne Hospital, New Zealand 2003

Thirty eight subjects previously diagnosed with asthma by their GP and using moderate to high doses of medication participated in the trial. All subjects were between the ages of 18 and 70 years.

Participants completed a diary card recording symptoms and medication use for four weeks before the trial. Subjects were then paired on asthma severity and allocated to either the control or the Buteyko group by a computer generated list.

The Buteyko group were taught exercises aimed at promoting hypoventilation (reduced volume breathing).

General asthma education and relaxation techniques currently employed by Gisborne Hospital were taught to the control group.

During the trial, each participant completed diary cards at six week, three month and six month assessments. In order to remove any contact bias, tutor contact in both groups following the trial was equal and minimal.

Trial results

Medication usage after six months

Buteyko Group

Average reduction in reliever use: 85%
Average reduction in inhaled steroid use: 50%

Control Group

Average reduction in reliever use: 37%
Average change in inhaled steroid use: 1% increase

The Buteyko group had clinically significant difference in their use of reliever medication and inhaled steroid use 'without negative impact on measures of lung function and with no apparent adverse effects'.[4]

Conclusion

The New Zealand Medical Journal commented with the following:

'The ability to produce marked reductions in asthma-drug utilisation suggests that the pharmaco-economic implications of BBT (Buteyko Breathing Technique) merit further study. Clarification of the mechanism(s) underlying the effectiveness of BBT is a further goal, given that BBT appears to represent a safe, efficacious alternative for the treatment of asthma.'

[For a more detailed synopsis of the trial, please refer to *The New Zealand Medical Journal*. Vol 116. No 1187]

house of commons debate

June 25th, 2002

During a debate in the British House of Commons, Westminster, London, on June 25th, 2000, **Mrs Anne Campbell** (Cambridge) commented as follows:

'It is time we admitted that the current treatments appear to be making us worse, not better, and I want to take a look at the possible causes and treatment of asthma. I shall describe the work done by a Russian doctor, Konstantin Buteyko, in the 1960s; it attempted to explain why people get asthma, and offered a management regime for the disease. Dr Buteyko's methods were practised widely in Russia in the 1980s, and that may still be the case. They spread to Australia when an Australian doctor suffered an asthma attack while visiting Russia. He was admitted to hospital and was taught the Buteyko Method for controlling his symptoms. He was so impressed that he took the method back to Australia, and it is now taught there and in New Zealand.

Buteyko blames hyperventilation for a number of civilisation-induced diseases. We all hyperventilate at times of stress.

There are some well-documented cases of people who have been helped by the technique. I understand that

Jonathan Aitken, when he was Chief Secretary to the Treasury, received treatment from a Buteyko practitioner in London. His asthma was moderately severe, but over a course of consultations and home visits he made a dramatic recovery. A newspaper article quoted him as saying: 'I have tried plenty of treatments, but this is the only one that has really worked. I think it is a remarkable one that could help many people.'

Con Barrell, a member of the New Zealand All-Black team, said after his treatment: 'I sleep better, my pulse rate has dropped 10–12 beats on a regular basis and I feel well. This has been a big help to me as a professional and personally. I recommend asthmatics try it – things can only get better.'

As someone who has suffered from asthma for 40 years and whose condition would have been previously described as moderate, I have given the Buteyko technique a try myself. I started with a home education pack, as described on the website, www.buteyko.co.nz. Even self-teaching is effective, as by day five I had reduced the number of times I took my reliever medication from four or five times a day to very occasional use. Later I went on a course run by a qualified Buteyko practitioner. As I continued, I discovered to my delight that the asthma symptoms were rapidly reduced. I sleep better and have more energy than I can ever remember.

What I really regret is that no one told me about the method before. This year I have not suffered from any hay fever, except for a very occasional sneeze, and I wish that someone had told me about the technique some time ago. Alone, I could have saved the National Health Service hundreds of pounds worth of medication and myself a lot of needless discomfort. However, the Minister, whom I am happy to welcome to the Front Bench, will be less impressed by anecdote than by medical trials. Unfortunately, there is little evidence to quote so far.

Later during the same debate, the same speaker had this to contribute:

'In referring to the effectiveness of the Buteyko Method, the National Asthma Campaign remarks on its website: 'Lack of published research makes it difficult to reach a conclusion on its effectiveness.'

Buteyko himself conducted a trial in Russia, but the results were considered to be too good, and were not believed for many years.

In December 1998 a paper by Bowler, Green and Mitchell was published in *Alternative Medicine*, in Australia. The paper was called *Buteyko breathing techniques in asthma: a blinded randomised trial*. The trial compared the effect of the Buteyko Breathing technique with a control group in thirty-nine subjects with asthma. The control group was given instruction in general asthma education, relaxation techniques and abdominal breathing exercises. The experimenters looked at medication use, peak flow and quality of life, among other factors.

After three months, the subjects assigned to the Buteyko group had reduced their reliever medication by 904 micrograms, whereas the control group had a reduction of 57 micrograms – a highly significant result at the 0.2 per cent level of significance. There was also a reduction in inhaled steroid use by the Buteyko subjects, although the sample sizes were too small for that to be statistically significant.

Similarly and more importantly, perhaps from my point of view, there was a trend towards greater improvement in the mean quality of life scores of the Buteyko group. I certainly think that if someone can have uninterrupted sleep, feel better and have more energy, it is worth a great deal to that individual.

I should like to mention Jill McGowan, who was awarded the Carer of the Year award at the Pride of Britain Awards 2002. She knows a lot about asthma because she has the condition herself, and is also a nurse who has worked for many years helping other asthmatics. Like many others who have followed the course, she stopped needing her inhaler within twenty-four hours.

Jill is also a university lecturer with the skills to look into the theory behind Buteyko. When she decided that the method had merit, she was amazed to find that it was not more widely researched. She applied to universities for grants to allow her to fund a pilot study. When they turned her down, she sold her house and used the £55,000 proceeds to pay for the study herself.

The pilot study has shown excellent results – a more than ninety per cent reduction in reliever medication in the first few weeks. Because of those results, a two-year clinical study of 600 asthma sufferers is under way. Jill is also helping to pay for that work by donating three-quarters of her salary. That is real dedication. She hopes that the clinical study will prove the benefits of the Buteyko technique, so that one day it can become available to all on the NHS.

I very much hope that as a result of this adjournment debate, my Honourable Friend will ask the Chief Medical

Officer to examine the available evidence. In particular, I would ask him to consider the preliminary evidence from the Scottish trial, and to have further trials conducted to ascertain the method's efficacy in the UK. Let me stress that the technique that I have described does not constitute alternative medicine – a term normally used to describe techniques that sometimes succeed, although no-one can quite work out why. The Buteyko technique was derived from research carried out by Konstantin Buteyko, who devised a programme from his theory. The fact that it has worked for me, as well as for many others, must suggest that at the very least it is worth investigating further. I hope that the Minister will respond positively to that suggestion.

Konstantin Pavlovich Buteyko

Konstantin Pavlovich Buteyko was born near Kiev in The Ukraine on January 27th, 1923. This simple yet extraordinary man devoted his life to studying the human organism and made one of the most profound discoveries in the history of medicine.

Buteyko commenced his medical training in Russia in 1946 at the First Medical Institute of Moscow. Part of one of his practical assignments involved monitoring the breathing of terminally ill patients prior to death. After hundreds of hours spent observing and recording breathing patterns, he was able to predict with accuracy, often to the minute, the time of death of each patient. Each patient's breathing increased as their condition deteriorated and as they approached death.

While at University Buteyko was diagnosed as suffering from severe hypertension, which gave him a life expectancy of just 12 months. Under the guidance of his tutors Buteyko researched his illness in depth although it seemed that there was very little that he could do to reverse it.

On October 7th, 1952 after majoring in clinical therapy, he began to wonder whether the cause of his condition, which was going from bad to worse, might be his deep breathing. He checked this by reducing his breathing. Within minutes his headache, the pain in his right kidney and his heartache ceased. To confirm his discovery, he took five deep breaths and the pain returned. He again reversed his deep breathing and the pain disappeared.

He did not appreciate it at the time, but this was one of the greatest, although as yet largely unacknowledged, medical discoveries of the twentieth century. Buteyko established that breathing, so vital in sustaining life, can not be alone the cure but also, amazingly, the cause of so many diseases of civilisation.

Buteyko's next step was to seek out the theory which would support his discovery. The data then available (in 1952) from authors such as Holden, Priestly, Henderson, De Costa, Werigo, and Bohr, seemed to confirm his hypothesis. It was known at that time that exhaling carbon dioxide by deep breathing resulted in spasms which decreased the supply of oxygen to vital organs, including the brain thus making one breathe deeper again. This completed a vicious circle.

Buteyko measured the breathing patterns of patients suffering from asthma, but he also included in his research sufferers from other ailments and found in many cases that they too hyperventilated between attacks. After many years research, he went on to work on the theoretical aspects of his discovery at the Central and Lenin Medical Libraries. He devised a programme to measure breathing and also a method of reconditioning patients' breathing to normal levels. This involved:

1. Switching from mouth breathing to nasal breathing.
2. Relaxation of the diaphragm until an air shortage is felt.

3. Small lifestyle changes are necessary to assist with this, thus commencing the road to full recovery.

Buteyko received a cold reception from the medical establishment at the time. In order to have his discovery accepted he commenced clinical research on a mixed group of two hundred people – some sick and some healthy, in 1959. On January 11th, 1960 he demonstrated to the Scientific Forum at the Institute the correlation between depth of breathing, carbon dioxide levels in the body and state of health.

However, for many of his colleagues Dr Buteyko offered too great a challenge to many of the theories upon which medicine was based. Surely illness, for which the conventional medical remedy was surgery and/or extensive medication, could not be dealt with simply by a change in breathing. Yet this was exactly what Buteyko demonstrated. And while not receiving outright acceptance, Buteyko did gain the temporary support of Professor Meshalkin, the chairman of the Forum, in enabling the research to continue.

In the years that followed, Buteyko continued his research, assisted by a team of two hundred qualified medical personnel and using the most up to date technology. By 1967 over one thousand patients with asthma, and other illnesses, had recovered from their conditions using his methods.

Unfortunately Professor Meshalkin continually refused to allow a scientific trial of the Buteyko Method. Later, this was followed by closure of his laboratory and outright repression. There were even reports of attempts on his life by mysterious car accidents and food poisoning.

However in January 1968, following growing public support, Health Minister Academician Petrovsky, promised that he would endorse acceptance of the Buteyko Method as an acceptable standard medical practice if Buteyko could demonstrate an eighty per cent success rate with patients. This was to be based on scientific evaluation of severe cases which were not treatable by conventional health management. Forty-six patients were taught his method and the results were astounding: one hundred per cent of the patients were officially diagnosed as cured. However in an extraordinary development and for no reason that can be established, falsified results were forwarded to the Minister. This subsequently resulted in the closure of Buteyko's laboratory.

But the good doctor persevered and, in April 1980, following trials in Leningrad and at the First Moscow Institute of Pediatric Diseases, the Buteyko Breathing Method was officially acknowledged as having a one hundred per cent success rate. This research was directed by the Soviet Ministry's Committee for Science and Technology.

The USSR Committee on Inventions and Discoveries formally acknowledged Buteyko's discovery in 1983 and issued the patent entitled 'The method of treatment of hypocapnia', (Authors certificate No. 1067640 issued on September 15th, 1983). Interestingly, the date of the discovery as listed in the document was backdated to January 29th, 1962. His discovery was officially recognised twenty years after it had been made.

Over two hundred medical professionals teach this therapy at present from centres located in major towns throughout Russia. Buteyko wrote over fifty scientific publications detailing the relationship between respiration and carbon dioxide and at least five Ph.D. dissertations were written by his colleagues. The basis of the Buteyko Breathing Method detailing the relationship between carbon dioxide and breath holding-time forms part of medical curriculum at Universities.

During my time at the Buteyko Clinic in Moscow, Professor Buteyko's health was failing due to a very serious car accident in which he had been involved ten years previously. Although he visited the clinic regularly, he had retired at that time and instead devoted his mind to matters of a more spiritual nature.

On Friday, May 2nd 2003 at 4.05 p.m. (Moscow time), Professor Buteyko parted from this world with some very deep inspirations. His death came as quite a shock to the many people around the world who had experienced excellent health as a result of his life's work. His wish was to be buried in the country of his birth, the Ukraine. His resting place is in Feodosia in the Crimea, Ukraine.

His memory will live on and I feel will grow in momentum as more and more people hear about his discovery.

In 1990 the Buteyko Method was brought outside Russia to Australia by Sasha Stalmatski. Working from his apartment in Sydney, he began by treating only Russian friends and family. Gradually over the years more people learned of this new method and media coverage in both newspapers and TV helped to increase awareness. In 1995 Stalmatski brought this method to the UK and, for a number of years, it has been practised at the famous Hale Clinic (opened in 1988 by Prince Charles).

It is estimated that over the past five decades more than 100,000 people have learned and applied this therapy in Russia, some 25,000 in Australia and New Zealand, and many thousands in the UK.

Buteyko's Method challenges the belief that overbreathing is beneficial and also uncovers many causes of illness unexplained by modern medicine. It seems extraordinary that modern medicine, with all its research and resources, human, technical and scientific, has continually failed to verify the link between overbreathing and various medical conditions, notably asthma.

The efforts which Buteyko had to make to have his discovery recognised also seem to indicate an unwillingness on the part of the medical community to accept discoveries not pharmaceutically based – in part perhaps because they challenge long standing and sincerely held beliefs.

My own belief is that Buteyko will in time gain full acceptance from the medical community, although it may take some years. This will happen mainly as a result of the growing number of people worldwide who are experiencing a life changing improvement in health within a relatively short period of time. These people will be the most ardent followers of Buteyko, and I consider myself to be part of this group. It is our own direct experience that compels us to tell people, and thus spread the word, about the method of this extraordinary doctor. The quicker this can be accomplished, the greater the contribution that Buteyko's discovery will make to the health of mankind generally and asthma sufferers in particular.

references

Chapter 1: Asthma for Beginners

1. WHO Fact Sheet No. 206, revised January 2000
2. National Centre for Health Statistics: National Health Survey 2001
3. National Asthma Campaign www.asthma.org.uk - Asthma Audit 2001 Summary
4. Commonwealth Dept of Health and Aging 9 May 2003
5. Asthma Society of Ireland 2004

Chapter 2: How is Your Breathing?

1. Johnson BD, Scanlon PD, Beck KC; 'Regulation of ventilatory capacity during exercise in asthmatics', *J Appl Physiol*, 1995 Sep 79(3) 892–901
2. Bowler SD, Green A, Mitchell CA; 'Buteyko breathing techniques in asthma, a blinded randomised controlled trial', *Med J of Australia*, 1998 169, 575–578
3. McFadden ER, Lyons HA; 'Arterial Blood gases in asthma', *The New England Journal of Medicine*, 1968 May 9, 278 (19) 1027–1032

4. Gulati MS, Grewal N, Kaur A; 'A comparative study of effects of mouth breathing and normal breathing on gingival health in children', *J Indian Soc Pedod Prev Dent.*, 1998 Sep;16(3):72–83

Chapter 4: Make Correct Breathing a Habit

1. Lingoes G, Morton JAR, Henry RLA; 'Mirth-triggered asthma: Is laughter really the best medicine?', *Pediatr Pulmonol.*, August 2003, 36(2):107–12
2. Young E; 'Laughter is major asthma trigger', *New Scientist*; March 28th, 2002
3. Pagán Westphal S; 'Bed-wetters could breathe easier', *New Scientist*, July, 30th, 2003, 19:00
4. Peter J Barnes & Michael T Newhouse, *Conquering Asthma*
5. Dr John McKenna, *Natural Alternatives to Antibiotics*
6. Singh V, Wisniewski A, Britton J, Tattersfield A; 'Effect of Yoga breathing exercises (pranayama) on airway reactivity in subjects with asthma', *The Lancet*, 1990, volume 335 1381–83

Chapter 5: Breathe Right During Physical Activity

1. Clark C, Cochrane L; 'Assessment of work performance in asthma for determination of cardiorespiratory fitness and training capacity', *Thorax*, 1988; 43: 745–749
2. Garfinkel S, Kersten S, Chapman K, Rebuck A; 'Physiologic and nonphysiologic determinants of aerobic fitness in mild to moderate asthma', *American Review of Respiratory Disease*, 1992; 145; 741–745

3. Orenstein DM, Reed ME, Grogan Jr. FT, Crawford LV; 'Exercise conditioning in children with asthma', *The Journal of Pediatrics*, 1985; 106:556–560

4. Counil FP, Varray A, Matecki S, Beurey A, Marchal P, Voisin M, Prefaut C; 'Training of aerobic and anaerobic fitness in children with asthma', *J Pediatr*, February 2003;142(2):179–84

5. Gotshall RW; 'Exercise-induced bronchoconstriction', *Drugs*, 2002; 62(12):1725–39

6. Anderson S, Holzer K; 'Exercise-induced asthma: Is it the right diagnosis in elite athletes?', *Journal Allergy Clin. Immunol*, 2000; 106:419–28

7. Larsson K, Ohlsen P, Larsson L, et al.; 'High prevalence of asthma in cross country skiers', *BMJ*, 1993; 307: 1326–1329

8. Sue-Chu M, Larrson L, Bjermer L; 'Prevalence of asthma in young cross country skiers in central Scandinavia; a difference between Norway and Sweden', *Respir Med*, 1996; 90:99–105

9. Wilber RL, Rundell KW, Szmedra L, Jenkinson DM, Im J, Drake SD; 'Incidence of exercise-induced bronchospasm in Olympic winter sport athletes', *Med Sci Sports Exerc.*, April 2000; 32(4):732–7

10. Donnelly PM; 'Exercise-induced asthma: The protective role of CO_2 during swimming', *The Lancet*, January 1991; 337(8734): 179–80

11. Wardell CP, Isbister C; 'A swimming program for children with asthma: Does it improve their quality of life?', *MJA*, 2000; 173: 647–648

12. Smith E, Mahony N, Donne B, O'Brien M; 'Prevalence of obstructive airflow limitation in Irish collegiate athletes', *Ir J Med Sci.*, October–December 2002;171(4):202–5

Chapter 6: Food That Helps, Food That Hurts

1. Denny SI, Thompson RL, Margetts BM; 'Dietary factors in the pathogenesis of asthma and chronic obstructive pulmonary disease', *Curr Allergy Asthma Rep.*, 2003 Mar;3(2):130–6

2. John Kenneth Galbraith, *The Affluent Society*

3. Huang SL, Lin KC, Pan WH; 'Dietary factors associated with physician-diagnosed asthma and allergic rhinitis in teenagers: analyses of the first Nutrition and Health Survey in Taiwan', *Clin Exp Allergy.*, 2001 Feb;31(2):259–64

4. W M Fox, *Asthma: Is your suffering really necessary?* Hale London.

5. Leon Chatow, *Stone Age Diet, the Natural Way to Eat*

6. Versluis RG, *et al*; 'Prevalence of osteoporosis in postmenopausal women in family practice' [Article in Dutch], *Ned Tijdschr Geneeskd*, 1999 Jan 2;143(1):20–4

7. Dr Weston Price, *Nutrition and Physical Degeneration*

8. Professor Jonathan Brostoff, *Asthma: The Complete Guide*

9. Brunner EH, *et al*; 'Effect of parenteral magnesium on pulmonary function, plasma C-amp, and histamine in bronchial asthma', *Journal Asthma*, 22 (1985): 3

10. Okayama H, *et al*; 'Bronchodilating effect of intravenous magnesium sulphate in bronchial asthma', *Journal of the American Medical Association*, 257 (1987): 1076

11. Skobeloff EM, *et al;* 'Intravenous magnesium sulphate for the treatment of acute asthma in the emergency department', *Journal of the American Medical Association,* 282 (1989): 1210

12. Wei W, Franz KB; 'A synergism of antigen challenge and severe magnesium deficiency on blood and urinary histamine levels in rats', *Journal of the American College of Nutrition,* 9.6 (1990): 616–22

13. Hill J, Micklewright A, Lewis S, *et al;* 'Investigation of short term change in dietary magnesium intake in asthma', *Eur Respi Journal,* 1997 p2225

14. Dominguez LJ, Barbagallo M, Di Lorenzo G, Drago A, Scola S, Morici G, Caruso C; 'Bronchial reactivity and intracellular magnesium: a possible mechanism for the bronchodilating effects of magnesium in asthma', *Clin Sci* (London), 1998 Aug;95(2):137–42

15. Habya MM, Peatb JK, Marksc GB, Woolcockc AJ, Leederd SR; 'Asthma in preschool children: prevalence and risk factors', *Thorax,* August 2001;56:589–595

16. Simopoulos AP; 'Omega-3 Fatty Acids in Inflammation and Autoimmune Diseases', *Journal of the American College of Nutrition,* 2002 Vol. 21, No. 6, 495–505

17. Mihrshahi S, Peat JK, Marks GB, Mellis CM, Tovey ER, Webb K, Britton WJ, Leeder SR; 'Eighteen month outcomes of house dust mite avoidance and dietary fatty acid modification in the Childhood Asthma Prevention Study (CAPS)', *J Allergy & Clin. Immunology,* 2003, 111(1), 162 8

18. Melshart D, Linde K, Worku F, *et al;* 'Immunomodulation with Echinacea – a systematic review of controlled clinical trials', *Phytomedicine,* 1994;1:245–54

19. Dorn M, Knick E, Lewith G; 'Placebo-controlled, double blind study of echinacea pallida redix in upper respiratory tract infections', *Comp Ther Med,* 1997; 5:40–2

20. Hoheisel O, Sandberg M, Bertram S, *et al;* 'Echinacea shortens the course of the common cold: a double blind placebo controlled clinical trial', *Eur J Clin Res,* 1997; 9:261–8

Chapter 7: What's Your Trigger?

1. Joseph KE, Adams CD, Cottrell L, Hogan MB, Wilson NW; 'Providing dust mite-proof covers improves adherence to dust mite control measures in children with mite allergy and asthma', *Ann Allergy Asthma Immunol,* May 2003; 90(5):550–3

2. Lee IS; 'Effect of bedding control on amount of house dust mite allergens, asthma symptoms, and peak expiratory flow rate', *Yonsei Med J,* April 30th, 2003; 44(2):313–22

3. von Mutius E, Weiland SK, Fritzsch C, Duhme H, Keil U; 'Increasing prevalence of hay fever and atopy among children in Leipzig, East Germany', *The Lancet,* March 21st, 1998;351(9106):862–6

4. Vander, Sherman, Luciano; *Human Physiology,* 1998; p463

Chapter 8: Know Your Medication

1. Soler M; 'Asthma therapy: are bronchodilators obsolete?' [Article in German], *Schweiz Med Wochenschr*, 1992 Mar 28;122(13):455–60

2. Peter J Barnes, Simon Godfrey; *Asthma Therapy*, 1998 p53

3. Lundback B, Alexander M, Day J, Hebert J, Holzer R, van Uffelen R, *et al*; 'Evaluation of fluticasone propionate (500 µg/day) administered either as a dry powder via diskhaler or pressurised inhaler and compared with beclomethasone dipropionate (1000 µg/day) administered by pressurised inhaler', *Respir Med*, 1993;87:609–620

4. Gustafsson P, Tsanakas J, Gold M, Primhak R, Radford M, Gillies E; 'Comparison of the efficacy and safety of inhaled fluticasone propionate 200 µg/day with inhaled beclomethasone dipropionate 400 µg/day in mild and moderate asthma', *Arch Dis Child*, 1993;19:206–211

5. Leblanc P, Mink S, Keistinen T, Saaelainen PA, Ringdal N, Payne SL; 'A comparison of fluticasone propionate 200 µg/day with beclomethasone dipropionate 400 µg/day in adult asthma', *Allergy*, 1994;49:380–385

6. Peter J Barnes, Simon Godfrey; *Asthma Therapy*, 1998, p49

7. 'The British Guidelines on Asthma Management', 1995 Review and Position Statement, *Thorax* 1997;52 (90001):S1–S20 (February)

8. Hancox RJ, Taylor DR; 'Long-acting beta-agonist treatment in patients with persistent asthma already receiving inhaled corticosteroids', *BioDrugs*, 2001;15(1):11–24

9. 'Are Asthma Drugs the Cure that kills?', *New Scientist*, 6th April 1991

10. Professor Jonathan Brostoff and Linda Gamlin; *Asthma: The Complete Guide*

11. Sears MR, Taylor DR; 'The beta 2-agonist controversy. Observations, explanations and relationship to asthma epidemiology', *Drug Saf.*, 1994 Oct;11(4):259–83

12. Sears MR; 'Changing patterns in asthma morbidity and mortality', *J Investig Allergol Clin Immunol.*, 1995 Mar–Apr;5(2):66–72

13. Habbick B, Baker MJ, McNutt M, Cockcroft DW; 'Recent trends in the use of inhaled beta 2-adrenergic agonists and inhaled corticosteroids in Saskatchewan', *CMAJ*, 1995 Nov 15;153(10):1437–43

14. Cookcroft DW, McParland CP, Britto SA, Swystun VA, Rutherford BC; 'Regular inhaled Salbutamol and airway responsiveness to allergen', *The Lancet*, Vol342, October 2, 1993

15. Hancox RJ, Subbarao P, Kamada D, Watson RM, Hargreave FE, Inman MD; 'Beta2-agonist tolerance and exercise-induced bronchospasm', *Am J Respir Crit Care Med.*, 2002 Apr 15;165(8):1068–70

16. Barg W, Obojski A, Panaszek B, Markowska-
Woyciechowska A, Wytrychowski K, Malolepszy J; 'Non-
compliance resulting in fatal asthmatic attack in a
27-year-old woman' [Article in Polish], *Pol Arch Med
Wewn.*, 2002 Dec;108(6):1199–1203

17. Hancox RJ, Subbarao P, Kamada D, Watson RM,
Hargreave FE, Inman MD; 'Beta2-agonist tolerance and
exercise-induced bronchospasm', *Am J Respir Crit Care
Med.*, 2002 Apr 15;165(8):1068–70

18. FDA website T03-06 23rd January 2003.

Chapter 9: How to Help Children and Teenagers

1. Gulati MS, Grewal N, Kaur A; 'A comparative study of
effects of mouth breathing and normal breathing on
gingival health in children', *J Indian Soc Pedod Prev Dent*,
September 1998; 16(3): 72–83

2. Gdalevich M,.Mimouni D, Mimouni M; 'Breast-feeding
and the risk of bronchial asthma in childhood: a
systematic review with meta-analysis of prospective
studies', *J Pediatric*, August 2001; 139(2): 261–6

3. Oddy WH, Holt PG, Sly PD, Read AW, Landau LI, Stanley
FJ, Kendall GE, Burton PR; 'Association between breast-
feeding and asthma in 6 year old children: findings of a
prospective birth cohort study', *BMJ*, September 25th,
1999; 319 (7213): 815–9

4. Oddy WH, 'Breastfeeding and asthma in children:
findings from a West Australian study', *Breastfeed Rev.*,
Mar 2000; 8(1): 5–11

5. Chulada PC, Arbes SJ Jr, Dunson D, Zeldin DC; 'Breast-feeding and the prevalence of asthma and wheeze in children: analyses from the Third National Health and Nutrition Examination Survey', *J Allergy Clin Immunol.*, February 2003; 111(2): 328–36, *1988–1994*

Chapter 10: Individual and National Goals

1. Peter J. Barnes and Simon Godfrey; *Asthma Therapy*; 1998; p49

2. *Asthma Costs Irish Health Care System a Staggering €463m per Annum* Pharmaceutical & Clinical News, *IMJ*; May 2003; Volume 96, No 5.

3. *QED*, BBC1, 9.30 p.m, Wednesday, August 19th, 1998.

Appendix 2: Hyperventilation and Asthma

1. Demeter SL, Cordasco EM; 'Hyperventilation Syndrome and Asthma', *The American Journal of Medicine*, December 1986, Volume 81, p989

2. van den Elshout FJJ, van Herwaarden CLA, Folgering HTM; 'Effects of hypercapnia and hypocapnia on respiratory resistance in normal and asthmatic subjects', *Thorax*, 1991; 46, 28–32

3. Sterling GM; 'The Mechanism of Bronchoconstriction due to hypocapnia in man', *Clin Sci*, 1968; 34, 277-285

4. Hibbert GA, Pilsbury DJ; 'Demonstration and treatment of hyperventilation causing asthma', *British Journal of Psychiatry*, 1988; 153, 687–689

5. Brown EB Jr; 'Physiological effects of hyperventilation', *The American Physiological Society*, vol 33; October 1953; p445–461

6. McFadden ER, Lyons HA; 'Arterial Blood gases in asthma', *The New England Journal of Medicine*, 1968 May 9, 278 (19) 1027–1032

7. Gilbert IA, Fouke JM, McFadden ER Jr; 'Intra-airway thermodynamics during exercise and hyperventilation in asthmatics', *J Appl Physiol.*, 64; 2167–2174, 1988

8. Gilbert IA, McFadden ER Jr., 'Airway cooling and rewarming. The second reaction sequence in exercise-induced asthma', *J Clin Invest.*, 90; 699–704, 1992

9. McFadden ER Jr, Pichurko BM; 'Intra-airway thermal profiles during exercise and hyperventilation in normal man', *J Clin Invest.*, 76; 1007–1010, 1985

10. Anderson S, Holzer K; 'Exercise-induced asthma: Is it the right diagnosis in elite athletes?', *Journal Allergy Clin. Immunol*, 2000; 106:419–28

11. Rosenthal RR; 'Simplified eucapnic voluntary hyperventilation challenge', *J Allergy Clin Immunol*; May 1984; 73(5 Pt 2):676–9

12. Ohtsuka A, Koyama S, Yashizawa T, Kikuchi H, Horie T; 'Bronchoconstriction in isocapnic hyperventilation-induced asthma' [Article in Japanese], *Nihon Kyobu Shikkan Gakkai Zasshi*, October 1990; 28(10):1332–7

13. Roach JM, Hurwitz KM, Argyros GJ, Eliasson AH, Phillips YY; 'Eucapnic voluntary hyperventilation as a bronchoprovocation technique. Comparison with methacholine inhalation in asthmatics', *Chest*; March 1994; 105(3):667–72l

14. Johnson BD, Scanlon PD, Beck KC; 'Regulation of ventilatory capacity during exercise in asthmatics', *J Appl Physiol*, September 1995; 79(3) 892–901

15. Bowler SD, Green A, Mitchell CA; 'Buteyko breathing techniques in asthma, a blinded randomised controlled trial', *Med J of Australia*, 1998, 169, 575–578

16. McFadden ER Jr, Pichurko BM; 'Intra-airway thermal profiles during exercise and hyperventilation in normal man', *J Clin Invest.*, 76; 1007–1010, 1985

17. Lingoes G, Morton JAR, Henry RLA; 'Mirth-triggered asthma: Is laughter really the best medicine?', *Pediatr Pulmonol*, August 2003; 36(2):107–12

18. Young E; 'Laughter is major asthma trigger', *New Scientist;* March 28th, 2002

19. Reggiani E, Marugo L, Delpino A, Piastra G, Chiodini G; 'A comparison of various exercise challenge tests on airway reactivity in atopical swimmers', *J Sports Med Phys Fitness*, 1988; 28:394–401

20. Cardain L, Stager J; 'Pulmonary structure and function in swimmers', *Sports med*, 1988; 6:271–78

21. Kohrt WM, Morgan DW, Bates B, Skiner JS; 'Physiological responses of tri athletes to maximal swimming, cycling and running', *Med Sci Sports Exercise*, 1987; 19: 51–55

Appendix 3: Controlled Buteyko Trials

1. *MJA* 1998; 169: 575-578. Simon D Bowler, Amanda Green and Charles A Mitchell

2. James Hooper, *The Buteyko Manual for Asthma*

3. *Australian Doctor*, 7 April 1995.

4. *The New Zealand Medical Journal*, Vol 116. No 1187

Additional References

1. Professor Jonathan Brostoff, *Asthma: The Complete Guide*
2. Teresa Hale, *Breathing Free*
3. Buteyko Support Group worldwide organized by Peter Kolb of Australia
4. Alexander Stalmatski, *Freedom from Asthma*
5. Artour Rakhimov Ph.D., *What Science and Professor Buteyko Teach Us About Breathing*
6. Dr Andrey Novozhilov, *Personal Correspondence*
7. Robert Fried Ph.D., *Breathe Well, Be Well*
8. Dr Paul J. Ameisen, *Every Breath You Take*
9. Echart Tolle, *The Power of Now*
10. Dinah Bradley, *Hyperventilation Syndrome*
11. Richard N. Firshien, *Reversing Asthma*
12. Dennis Lewis, *The Tao of Natural Breathing*

Diary of Progress (Adults Page 1)

Date												
Time												
Pulse												
CP												
RB 5 min												
CP												
RB 5 min												
CP												
RB 5 min												
CP												
RB 5 min												
CP												
Pulse												

CP means Control Pause. **RB 5 min** means reduced breathing for five minutes. Rest for one minute before taking CP.

Diary of Progress (Adults Page 2)

Date													
Time													
Pulse													
CP													
RB 5 min													
CP													
RB 5 min													
CP													
RB 5 min													
CP													
RB 5 min													
CP													
Pulse													

CP means Control Pause. **RB 5 min** means reduced breathing for five minutes. Rest for one minute before taking CP.

Diary of Progress (Adults Page 3)

Date													
Time													
Pulse													
CP													
RB 5 min													
CP													
RB 5 min													
CP													
RB 5 min													
CP													
RB 5 min													
CP													
Pulse													

CP means Control Pause. **RB 5 min** means reduced breathing for five minutes. Rest for one minute before taking CP.

Diary of Progress (Steps Page 1)

Date															
Time															
CP															
Steps															
Steps															
Steps															
CP															
Steps															
Steps															
Steps															
Mouse															
CP															

CP means Control Pause. **Mouse** means reduced breathing for 3–5 minutes, to 'breathe like a little mouse'.

Diary of Progress (Steps Page 2)

Date												
Time												
CP												
Steps												
Steps												
Steps												
CP												
Steps												
Steps												
Steps												
Mouse												
CP												

CP means Control Pause. **Mouse** means reduced breathing for 3–5 minutes, to 'breathe like a little mouse'.

Diary of Progress (Steps Page 3)

Date												
Time												
CP												
Steps												
Steps												
Steps												
CP												
Steps												
Steps												
Steps												
Mouse												
CP												

CP means Control Pause. **Mouse** means reduced breathing for 3–5 minutes, to 'breathe like a little mouse'.

index